PAIN

Nerves On Fire
Changing Neuropathic Pain

Jay Tracy, PA-C, PsyD, LP

Illustrations by

SYDNEY KLOSTER
DAR DAILY

ISBN-10: 1466476079
EAN-13: 9781466476073

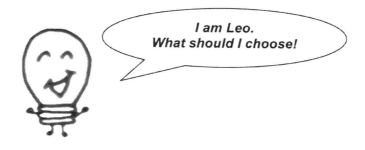

"Leo alight"

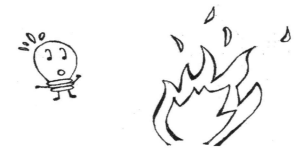

"Leo Enlightened"

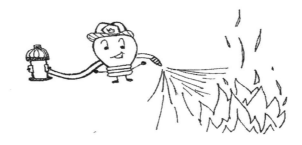

What can I do for myself?

Forward and Comments

More often than not, chronic pain patients are confused by what is happening to them, why they are not getting better, and why their medical providers do not seem to "get it." Significant others in the patient's life see the person's pain through the lens of acute pain instead of chronic pain. Acute pain, after all, gets better, and so should the person. If the person doesn't get better, there's an assumption that it must be "in his head." The chronic pain patient, thinking himself alone and misunderstood, often withdraws into himself and sometimes doubts his own sanity. It is here that depression and anxiety take their foothold.

It is in this very climate that this book is so valuable to those with chronic pain. It sorts through the confusion by looking at the complexities and chemistry of chronic pain, and, at the same time, clarifies these central issues with sensitivity, compassion, and humor. It is said that only a superb teacher who truly understands his subject can teach with simplicity, and this book answers that calling. Through the reading, the patient begins to understand what is happening to them physically, psychologically, and spiritually, and what aspects of functioning are preventing the person from living a full life. The sense of isolation starts to dissipate as the reader realizes his experience is not uncommon and he feels deeply understood and respected for the struggles involved in reclaiming one's life with chronic pain.

Anyone invested in truly understanding this complicated subject would benefit significantly from the material in this book and the masterful way in which it is presented.

Jacqueline Moeller, PsyD, LP

Clinical Psychologist

Courage Center

Golden Valley, Minnesota

Who are these patients who never get well? What is different about them? Why doesn't any treatment seem to work? And why do so many of them seem to simultaneously suffer multiple terrible disorders – pain, anxiety, depression, insomnia, fibromyalgia, migraine, TMJ, irritable bowel? These questions have plagued and frustrated patients and physicians for generations.

Now, in *Pain: Nerves On Fire, Changing Neuropathic Pain,* Dr. Jay Tracy has provided many of the answers we've needed. Written with the education-seeking chronic pain patient in mind, Dr. Tracy has assembled an unparalleled series of lessons on the causes and treatment of chronic pain syndromes from their microscopic molecular basis to the most advanced treatments being offered. The book's emphasis is on the physiology of the nervous system and its relationship to pain perception, cognition and ultimately, the experience of sensation. This is where Dr. Tracy's long career in treating these cases has led him – away from the quest for ever-more powerful medications and toward long-term life-management through a deep understanding of the pathophysiology of the disorders.

Pain: Nerves On Fire, Changing Neuropathic Pain, is not an easy book. It demands the reader's attention. It tells the complete story and will pay rich dividends to those who stick with it. For the sufferer of chronic pain, the most valuable return of all is a valid explanation of what to do when Medicine seemingly has failed and the pain won't go away. Finding and now sharing the meaning in that predicament is no small gift to those of us engaged in this struggle every day.

Brian S. Gould,
MD Staff Psychiatrist
Courage Center
Golden Valley, Minnesota

Dr. Tracy's book expertly synthesizes a difficult topic, mind-body interactions with chronic pain. This material serves to provide patients, clinicians, and students a paradigm and language to better understand human behavior and pain. The beauty of this book is that Dr. Tracy strikes a balance between technical descriptions and easily readable information. I strongly recommend this book for anyone afflicted or affected by chronic pain and particularly neuropathic pain.

Gary Goldetsky, PsyD, LP
Executive Vice President
On-Call Clinicians, Inc.
Clinical Health Psychologist
Courage Center
Golden Valley, Minnesota

Dr. Jay Tracy writes with insight, passion, experience, and clarity about subjects he loves, the brain, the body, and chronic pain. This book is a gateway for those who want to learn more about the complexities of chronic nerve-related pain.

Margaret Keller, RN, ACNS, BC
Clinical Nurse Specialist
Courage Center
Golden Valley, Minnesota

Neuropathic pain, while a very common problem, is an extremely complex physiologic phenomenon. Dr. Tracy's genius is his ability to translate our understanding of this condition into a model that is accessible to patients who do not have a medical back ground. The information is presented in a way that not only educates individuals about this condition, but provides options to address the problem from a holistic perspective, empowering them to take back some control of their lives. I would recommend this book not only to patients but also to health providers who often struggle with presenting information to their patients about this condition in a manner that is easily understandable.

Matthew Monsein, MD
Medical Director
Chronic Pain Rehabilitation Program
Courage Center Golden Valley, Minnesota

This is an awesome book. Dr. Jay Tracy describes neuropathic pain in such a way as to educate and empower professionals and lay persons alike. The book is written with compassion and respect for all who struggle with this diagnosis.

Patti Pribyl-Brown, BS, CTRS, CCM
Certified Case Manager
Chronic Pain Rehabilitation Program
Courage Center
Golden Valley, Minnesota

Pain and Suffering

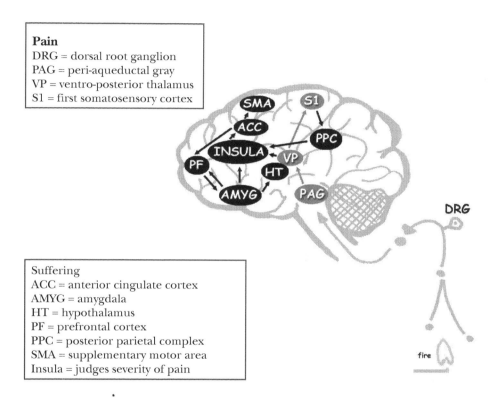

Pain
DRG = dorsal root ganglion
PAG = peri-aqueductal gray
VP = ventro-posterior thalamus
S1 = first somatosensory cortex

Suffering
ACC = anterior cingulate cortex
AMYG = amygdala
HT = hypothalamus
PF = prefrontal cortex
PPC = posterior parietal complex
SMA = supplementary motor area
Insula = judges severity of pain

This complex illustration is an attempt to show that the brain parts, networks, and pathways involved in pain are different than those involved in suffering. Pain is different than suffering. All of these parts and many others will be described as we progress through this book.

It might seem overwhelming to grasp the complicated and intricate concepts in this book. But this is the way pain is. It is very convoluted. There is no way to "just cut the nerve." When one method is used to block out pain the brain/body seems to compensate. It tries to find other ways to make sure one continues to feel pain. This book is an attempt to give the person who is suffering with chronic pain some understanding of what is normal and abnormal, and to give some hope in the whole medical and non-medical process.

Preface

It's a no brainer. Without the brain and the rest of the nervous system, we would not feel pain. No brain…no pain. This would not be good.

When it comes to pain, it seems that one of the functions of the nervous system is to protect us—to tell the truth about the threat of injury. We assume that pain has this purpose, to protect us from impending tissue damage. But what if something is wrong with the nervous system itself? What if the nervous system is not telling the truth?

Matt, a carpenter, accidentally cut off three of his fingers. He went through a fifteen-hour surgical repair of the fingers and hand. During that surgery his left leg was apparently resting in an odd position, and he developed a compartment syndrome of the left calf. This involved compression of nerves, blood vessels, and muscle inside the closed space of his terribly swollen calf. The fingers did not successfully reattach, but the hand healed without long-term pain. He subsequently had surgery on his leg. He also had diabetes, which hindered the healing of the leg. His leg became his main pain problem, which persisted for years. He described a symptom called **allodynia**: pain with even a very light touch. It hurt to put socks on. Cold worsened it. Heat helped slightly. He stated, "It is like numb and shooting, like asleep, and it hurts to step on it. Even the sheets of my bed hurt my foot. Sometimes it feels like *the nerves are on fire*. It is there all the time, like deep, hard pins and needles. It is healed but still hurts."

This pain persisted because there was something wrong with the nerves and the nervous system. It was not just a matter of "scar tissue on the nerves." There was nothing compressing the nerves that could be changed by surgical or interventional approaches. The nervous system itself had changed.

Bonnie suffered third degree full thickness burns to her legs, abdomen, and arms when she fell down the stairs while trying to discard burning grease in a fry pan. She was still experiencing pain with hypersensitivity years later, especially in her legs. Even a very light touch of the skin on her legs was painful. She described it as "a *burning like fire*, pinpricking, tingling, stabbing pain, worse when sitting in one place too long, worse with standing or exercise. It makes me irritable and grumpy. I was raised to be able to succeed even in hard times. I am having a lot of trouble with normal daily activities in work and school. I feel like I am being a baby about this hurting."

This ongoing pain is due to changes in the nervous system. These changes need not be permanent. Her emotional responses are biological, biochemical phenomena that can be changed. Much of what she experiences and how she responds can also be changed.

Karen had chronic daily headaches and deep, internal, constant anxiety for the past forty years. She also had degenerative disc disease in her neck and muscle tightness about her neck and shoulders. She was using 3 Vicodin per day but stated, "I don't want to become addicted." She was particularly **agoraphobic** (avoided going out for fear of having a panic attack) in the winter and had severe seasonal affective disorder. She jumped at any unusual sounds outside the office. Karen cried as she described many of her symptoms: "The headaches come on for no reason, as far as I can tell. Sometimes it feels like *my whole brain is on fire*. I completely shut down at times. I'm afraid to move my neck at times. I can't write or sit or read or even hold my grandchild." She related her problems to cruel and long-term abuse when she was a child. She was forced to do heavy and oppressive farm chores in the dark winter mornings without warm clothes or boots. "I had to carry large and overflowing buckets of icy water that sloshed over into my shoes," she stated. "I was punished for any spills. At that time I was young enough to be worried about the 'boogie man' in the dark. In reality, the boogie man was my father."

Karen's pain also persisted because there was something wrong with the nervous system. There was a significant and critical period of time when this young person's brain and nervous system were developing that she was inaccurately learning that fear and pain must go together. Parts of the nervous system developed in such a way that pain, anxiety, and fear became conjoined intensely and inappropriately.

Judy, a woman with *fibromyalgia* and **Raynaud's** (vascular constriction in her fingers when exposed to cold), described her sense of hypersensitivity to various stimuli throughout her life. She stated that when she was very young the tags in her clothes bothered her and she would ask her mother to cut them out. She described feeling very uncomfortable with anything tight around her waist. She always wondered why the pads on pens hurt the skin of her fingers and why the sounds from speakers on airplanes hurt her ears.

These symptoms are probably indicative of some type of pathology in the nervous system. But is this in the brain, the spinal cord, the peripheral nerves, or some combination of nervous system parts and networks? What might be the biological bases and biochemistry of such pathology?

In all of these cases, *neuropathic pain* is involved. Neuropathic pain refers to an experience associated with damage to the nervous system or dysfunction of the nervous system itself. The pain detectors and pain warning systems are malfunctioning. The person is experiencing pain when protection is not needed and there is no threat of impending tissue damage.

Imagine that the smoke detector in your home is damaged and oversensitive; it goes off when there is no smoke in the air. Imagine that the metal detector at the airport isn't sensitive enough and doesn't beep when you walk through with your artificial titanium hip replacement. Imagine that the pop machine rejects your perfectly good dollar bills. Imagine that it accepts counterfeit pieces of paper. Something is malfunctioning in these machines. Similarly, something can be malfunctioning in the nervous system as it experiences various stimuli and attempts to respond appropriately.

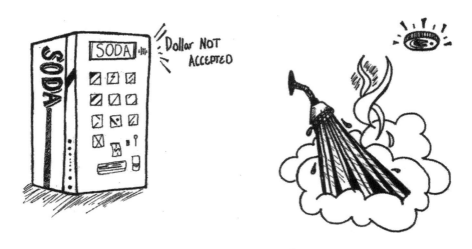

Neuropathic pain is a real medical problem, but it doesn't show up well on tests. If something doesn't show up on tests, there are many people, even medical people, who will believe that the problem does not exist. Sometimes patients are treated as though the problem is psychological or imaginary. Typically, this doesn't help.

Neuropathic pain is very often a long-term problem. Our society in general is quite intolerant of long-term problems. Patients and families can hardly understand why these problems cannot be found and fixed. A patient stated, "They put a man on the moon in 1969, for heaven's sake. Why can't they just fix this problem?" Neuropathic pain is real, but it is not easily understood or fixed.

Painful messages might not be telling the whole truth. The court testimony of a chemically impaired witness of a crime might not be totally reliable or accurate. With respect to neuropathic pain, the information about the painful stimulus and experience may not be totally accurate either.

What Could Go Wrong?

The damage that can occur in the nervous system may involve any of several parts of the nervous system. It may involve the small nerve endings at the site of injury, the nerve fibers that carry messages from the nerve endings to the spinal cord, the neurons and chemicals of the spinal cord that normally transmit messages up to the brain or down from the brain. It may involve damage to the part of the nervous system that normally understands, interprets, and responds to the meaning of the painful experience—the brain itself.

Understanding pain, neuropathic pain, and particularly pain that doesn't show up on tests, is very difficult…essentially impossible, really. It is more than just pain. It is often suffering as well. Pain is stressful and can have deleterious effects on the person experiencing it. The effects, the stress and strain of the pain, may be worse than the pain itself. The line from *My Fair Lady* by Alan J. Lerner and Frederick Lowe, "the rain in Spain stays mainly in the plain," can be modified to "the strain of pain lies mainly in the brain."

We can hardly understand some of the details of what is normal in the nervous system and the body, much less what really happens when things are abnormal. Without understanding these issues, how can we understand what to do about them or what to expect in the long-run?

Doctors make a lot of educated guesses. They attempt to help patients understand at least something because lack of information leads to fear of the unknown. Fear can make pain worse. Medical professionals try to describe things in terms that make sense to the patient and their loved ones. More information and knowledge can lead to less fear of the unknown.

So, What Can You Do About It?

If your medical professionals cannot make the problems go away, or even explain things in understandable terms, then start by learning as much as you can about your pain. Information may help you better understand why your symptoms are what they are, and why your doctor recommends various treatment approaches. That knowledge may help you understand what to expect for the future, help prevent or deal better with flare-ups or exacerbations of pain, give you the beginnings of a sense of control, and help you realistically focus on what can and cannot be done. You may waste less time, energy, and resources on approaches that will either not work, or only give you very temporary relief. The pain and its effects can take away your sense of control, power, and self-efficacy. It has been said that knowledge is power. When dealing with pain, this is true.

1. *Knowledge and understanding may lessen fear of the unknown.*
2. *Knowledge may help you understand more about why your doctor recommends various treatment approaches.*
3. *Knowledge may help you understand what to expect for the future.*
4. *Knowledge may help to prevent or deal better with flare-ups or exacerbations of pain or other problems.*
5. *Knowledge may give you the beginnings of a sense of control and help you realistically focus on what can and cannot be done.*

This book attempts to describe some of these complex issues about long-term pain, neuropathic pain, what is normal, what is abnormal, what to do about it, and what to expect. The intent is to give clear information about what is understood so far, and to lessen pain and the effects of pain in the lives of those who might appreciate this information. This book is a guide to better understand and change the clinical and personal experiences of neuropathic pain.

More information and knowledge can lead to less fear of the unknown.

Dedication

This book is dedicated to the patients and their families for their courageous efforts to improve their own and each other's very difficult situations.

Acknowledgements

Special thanks go to:

Ralph E. McKinney, Ph.D., L.P., my friend and mentor, who continues to teach me, through his life and example, how to really care for people and give them power in creative, enjoyable, and meaningful ways.

Matthew Monsein, MD, for his care and compassion when working with the patients and their complex situations.

Gary Goldetsky, PsyD, LP, for his friendship, editing, and encouragement in many ways.

Margaret Keller, RN, CNS, for her editing, inspired suggestions, and her kindness and compassion as she cares for patients.

Nancy Carlson, PsyD, LP, for her friendship and constant support.

Jacqueline Moeller, PsyD, LP, for her friendship, editing, and creative work with the patients.

Jim Koch, Ph.D., and all the various staff members of Bethel University in St. Paul, Minnesota, for allowing me to teach and learn about neuropsychology and the biological bases of behavior.

Lawrence J. Schut, MD, for many years of friendship and training in helping people control and deal better with chronic neurologic diseases, disabilities, and abilities. I thank him for helping me to understand that the "optimum level of functioning" (OLOF) is really a compromise between the patient's perspective and that of the professionals and others involved.

The staff of the Pain Management Program at Courage Center in Golden Valley, Minnesota.

The staff of the Pain Management Program at Sister Kenny Institute at Abbott Northwestern Hospital (which closed and moved to the Courage Center).

The doctors and staff at The Minneapolis Clinic of Neurology, Ltd., and my friends in the Rehabilitation Associates Pain Management Program, (This program operated from 1983-2001).

Dar Daily for his many hours of creative, artistic technical support, and his friendship.

Pat Daily for her editing, encouragement, and friendship.

Sydney Kloster for her joyful illustrations.

My daughters, Lisa and Megan, and son, Jason, and their spouses and children for their love.

And to my wife, Susan, for everything.

Table of Contents

Part 2: Beyond the Basics

Part 3: Pain Problems / Life Solutions

Introduction

"Absence of proof is not proof of absence."
CANDACE B. PERT. PH.D.,
MOLECULES OF EMOTION, P. 222

"In the shower it feels like I'm being hit by rock salt."
PATIENT

For Confused Patients Seeking Knowledge

You are suffering with long-term pain. You have seen many doctors, tried many treatments, and have only experienced temporary relief. Test results have been normal or have not really answered the questions you have been asking. The results may not have addressed the issues that are of most concern to you. You are confused and unclear about your diagnosis, treatment options, and expectations for the future. You are anxious, depressed, worried, frustrated, angry, and afraid. You've been told many things, many of which sound very complicated and unclear. To a certain extent, it seems that some people think the problem is imaginary, psychological, or all in your head. You just want to get fixed.

You understand that there is some structural problem, some anatomical pathology, or something wrong in your body. It may be in your muscles, ligaments, tendons, joints, bones, discs, fascia, nerves, or some other part of your body that is not functioning normally at this time. The specific structural, anatomical pathology has not shown up clearly on the tests and you are confused about this. You wonder if the doctors really know what is wrong with you. They only have so many tools to figure it out. One is your history. This is the information you are able to state to the doctor or what you tell the doctor about your symptoms and situation. Next is the examination, which involves only what the doctors can actually physically find with their own five senses. The third is the ancillary tests: x-rays, MRIs, blood tests, urine tests, etc.

In the end, the doctor may or may not have a clear understanding of what is wrong in your body. The doctor may or may not explain it to you in language you can understand. To you the information may still be very unclear.

The doctor may speak to you in generalities about long-term pain, the brain, the spinal cord, and biochemistry. You may hear or read about recent research in these areas. You may learn that the chemistry of pain is extremely complex and confusing. Without training and experience it is difficult to understand what is normal, much less what is abnormal.

The medical profession has known for quite some time that pain is more complicated than simple anatomy and physiology. It is known that long-term pain can cause actual anatomical, physiologic, and biochemical changes in the brain, spinal cord, and other parts and networks of the nervous system. The nervous system actually changes when bombarded by long-term pain. Taking an MRI of the brain or spinal cord experiencing painful messages might be like taking a picture of your computer when it is functioning incorrectly. It may *look* just fine but it might not be *working* correctly.

When a person experiences pain for a long time, there are changes that occur throughout the nervous system. This is like the wires in the walls of a house getting hot when the demand for electricity is beyond the capability of the electrical wiring system. If there is excess demand on the electrical system, or if the circuit breakers do not work, the wires might actually be damaged. They might become hot and cause a fire. The changes in the nervous system of a person experiencing long-term pain may aggravate and worsen a painful experience. The changes in the nervous system may cause many other sensations, perceptions, and responses as well.

You may have heard about conditions such as fibromyalgia, chronic fatigue syndrome, various sleep disorders, different types of headaches, myofascial pain or ongoing muscle tightness, arthritic and inflammatory diseases, anxiety and stress disorders, depression and other mood disorders, chemical dependency disorders, addiction, tolerance, and withdrawal. Even though these are all different conditions, they have underlying neurobiological similarities.

It is known that long-term pain can cause actual anatomical, physiologic, and biochemical changes in the brain, spinal cord, and other parts and networks of the nervous system.

Pain and Suffering

"Pain is inevitable. Suffering is optional."
   DALAI LAMA

"We are not cars. There is always going to be a psychological component."
   PATIENT.

"Sometimes the mental anguish far outweighs the physical pain."
   PATIENT.

What evidence exists for these statements? There are thousands of brain and nervous system parts, all of which constantly interact with each other and the body. They use millions of various networks and pathways, much like highways, county roads, city streets, and footpaths connecting various communities across a nation.

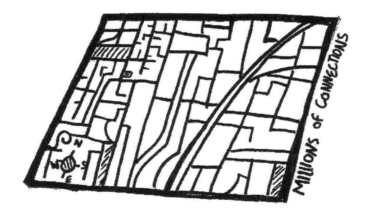

When pain is experienced, there are messages carried from one place to another using these various networks and pathways.

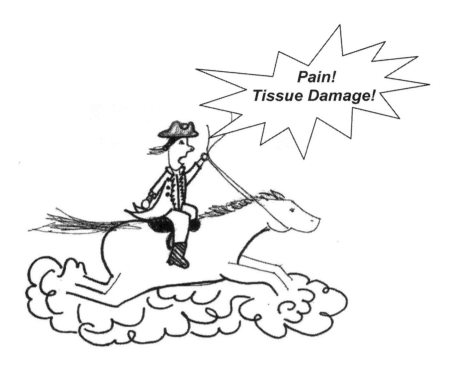

Imagine certain towns and cities that are specialized to experience painful messages and warn the nation about impending dangers, like a homeland security system. Various nerves, nerve endings, nerve wires, bundles of nerves throughout the body, the spinal cord, and the brain are specialized to send and receive painful messages. These messages occur when the nerves are stimulated by potential or actual tissue damage. This is true in all animals.

Pain and Suffering

Pain
DRG = dorsal root ganglion
PAG = peri-aqueductal gray
VP = ventro-posterior thalamus
S1 = first somatosensory cortex

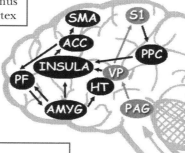

Suffering
ACC = anterior cingulate cortex
AMYG = amygdala
HT = hypothalamus
PF = prefrontal cortex
PPC = posterior parietal complex
SMA = supplementary motor area
Insula = judges severity of pain

The Brain In Pain

The *lighter* pathway represents the message of *pain* entering the spinal cord from a painful site. If your finger is burned by a flame, pain receptors in the skin of your finger pick up the painful messages. Then the messages travel up certain fibers or wires in your hand and arm, called ***A-delta*** and ***C fibers,*** that take the messages from the fingertip and bring it to the ***dorsal root ganglion (DRG)*** near the spinal cord. The dorsal root ganglion is a bundle of nerve cell bodies near the back side of the spinal cord. The painful messages go from there and enter the back side of the spinal cord called the ***dorsal horn***. The painful messages then travel up the spinal cord into the ***peri-aqueductal gray (PAG)***, then to the ***ventral posterior thalamus (VP)***, and up to the ***first somatosensory cortex (S1)***. This is essentially the simple, straight forward path of pain transmission from a painful stimulus to the places in the brain where the messages arrive and are perceived. The brain is where we really experience the pain. As stated earlier, "No brain… no pain."

A painful message can begin outside the body, such as with the flame, but can also begin from inside the body, such as with a tumor, ulcer, herniated disc, or many other medical problems. Many conditions such as arthritis, infections, vascular or blood vessel problems, various chemical problems in the body, degenerative diseases, musculoskeletal conditions, and even congenital conditions can be painful. Interestingly, even our own internal thoughts and feelings can cause or aggravate pain by changing the tension in the muscles or changing the electrical firing patterns in various parts and networks of the nervous system.

Even our own internal thoughts and feelings can cause or aggravate pain by changing the tension in the muscles or changing the electrical firing patterns in various parts and networks of the nervous system.

The Suffering Brain

"To live is to suffer. To survive is to find meaning in the suffering."
MAN'S SEARCH FOR MEANING
BY VICTOR FRANKL

"You can cripple yourself more in your mind."
PATIENT.

In human beings there are many brain parts, networks, and pathways in which thoughts and emotions about the painful experiences and their meanings may be very important. Pain is one thing, but suffering may involve ruminating about the past, thinking about what I used to be able to do, and worrying about the future, wondering how I am going to live with this the rest of my life. Consider our example of millions of nervous system networks and pathways being similar to highways and streets all across a nation. Imagine that there are certain towns and cities specialized to think about time—the past or the future. When these towns or cities are alerted and activated they transmit messages all over the country that have to do with time. If parts of the nervous system are designed to focus on the past or the future, then when they are stimulated the person will focus only on these issues. The person will ruminate about the past and worry about the future.

If there are parts of the nervous system stimulated to feel emotions when experiencing the pain, then the person may experience depression or anxiety and other feelings when contemplating the potential effects of long-term pain on life, work, play, and relationships, There are brain structures that do precisely these things. When these brain structures are stimulated, excited, recruited, and activated by the painful experience, the person focuses on all of these upsetting things. The pain becomes even more painful. The pain becomes "suffering."

The **darker** areas are involved in the **suffering** associated with the painful experience. These areas of the brain are also stimulated by the painful messages. In human beings, these areas are where the messages are assigned meanings. The meaning of the painful experience for the person becomes very important.

- "Will I be able to lift my grandchildren with this back pain the way it is?"
- "How will I be able to work with this neck pain?"
- "Do I have cancer?"
- "Is this degenerative disc disease going to progress and make me end up in a wheel chair?"
- "I used to be so active and enjoyed so many physical activities; now I can't do anything. My life is over."

For some people and situations pain may have a meaning that is good or beneficial. It may facilitate empathy. It may become something that gives strength or some other spiritual or socially constructive purpose. Sometimes it can be a useful positive experience. It is not always suffering. Sometimes it may be neither positive nor negative. It just is. But it is the brain that makes the difference. In reality, in human beings, pain involves thoughts, feelings, behaviors, and all the brain/body connections.

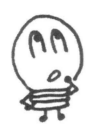

The strain of pain lies mainly in the brain.

In human beings there are many brain parts, networks, and pathways in which messages or emotions about the painful experiences and their meanings may be very important.

PART 1

THE BASICS

Atoms To Neurotransmitters

We begin by learning about the basics of the nervous system. This will set a foundation for understanding what might go wrong at times and the possible underlying pathology of the painful experience. That understanding will hopefully help us recognize what might be done to improve the situation.

Small parts of the brain/body connection

The brain/body connection is very complex. It involves all the individual parts, cells, fluids, chemicals, organs, and networks of the nervous system and the whole body. It comprises all of the many ways in which these parts and networks interact with each other. This includes how we think, feel, behave, and respond to various stimuli at various times and in various circumstances. This also incorporates how we relate to each other and even to the environment.

We need to understand what is *normal* in the brain/body in order to then understand what is *abnormal* when experiencing neuropathic or other types of pain. Even the basic terminology can be very confusing. One way to clarify much of this is to start with the smallest of structures and show how all the parts are built into the normally functioning human being. Once the basics are understood we might be better able to recognize what kinds of things can go wrong with the system that result in pain. We might also better understand what could be done to improve certain situations and what to expect for the future.

Let's start with atoms and build very quickly to the cells of the body, specifically the neurons of the nervous system, and the chemicals involved in the painful experience. The atom is one of the smallest structures. There are smaller *parts* of atoms, of course, but we will simply start with this extremely miniscule structure. If an atom was drawn to scale and the nucleus was the size of a ping-pong ball, we would need a screen a mile wide in order to display the electrons' orbits around the nucleus. Most of an atom is essentially empty space between the nucleus, which is made of protons and neutrons, and the swarm of orbiting electrons.

Atoms

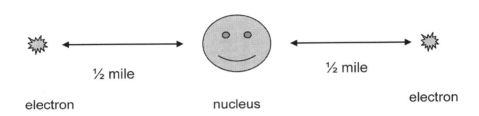

½ mile   ½ mile

electron   nucleus   electron

A molecule is the next structure of interest to us. A molecule is made up of many atoms that combine into organized clumps. Molecules are made from as few as two atoms or from as many as hundreds of millions of atoms. For example, two hydrogen atoms and one oxygen atom make up a molecule of water, H_2O, whereas various plant peptide hormones may have hundreds of millions of atoms in a single molecule.

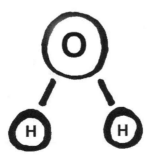

Molecules combine to become small particles that make up all living and non-living things. Of particular interest to us are the molecules called amino acids, each made from a few different atoms in various arrangements. There are twenty different amino acids. These are what make up the building blocks of all living things.

Amino Acids

Combinations of amino acids put together in a chain are called *peptides*. An example below might be the combination of two glycine molecules.

Peptide

Peptide Bond
A molecule of water is removed from two
glycine amino acids to form a peptide bond.

Many amino acid molecules strung together in a chain is called a *polypeptide*. If there are a hundred or fewer amino acids in a row, the polypeptide chain is simply called a peptide. If there are a hundred or greater (even many thousands) of amino acids in a chain, the structure is called a *protein*. Proteins make up many parts of the brain/body cells.

The *neurons* are the main cells of the nervous system. They are the main functional units of the nervous system. There are trillions of other cells in the body as well. Each cell has a membrane, like the skin of the cell. The membrane is riddled or embedded with large specially shaped clumps of protein that form channels or portals to allow other chemicals into and out of the cell. Imagine that each cell is like an apartment building and the channels or portals are like windows and doors in the building complex. These allow only certain people (or chemicals) to enter and exit.

POLYPEPTIDE

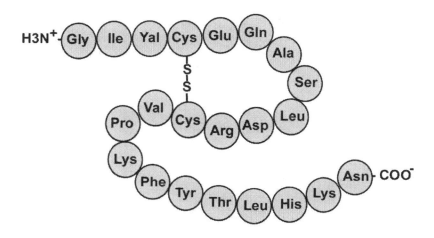

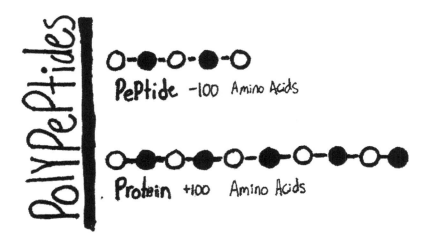

The neuron consists of mainly three parts: the cell body, called the *soma*, *dendrites* that basically receive messages from other neurons, and an *axon* which is a wire that carries messages away from the neuron and toward the next neuron in line. The axon has a *myelin*

sheath which is like insulation around a wire. Without the insulation, electric messages travel much more slowly down the wire. At the end of the axons there are *terminal buttons* or *axon terminals* where chemicals are excreted and go across the *synapse* to bind to and stimulate the next neuron in the line. Also, where the axon exits the cell body there is a structure called the *axon hillock*. This structure is very important. It makes decisions about sending messages from one neuron to the next. This will be described further in the next few pages.

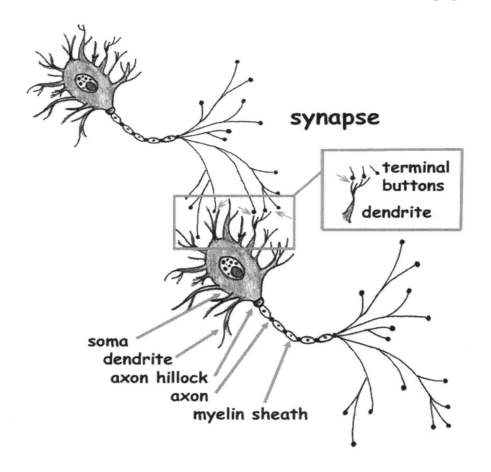

To gain perspective of the size of the various structures described one might consider a water droplet or a small pill or tablet of medication. Each is made of molecules which are extremely tiny. The number of water molecules in a drop of water is 18,400,000,000,000,000,000,000. This is 1.84×10 to the 21st power. When you take a small pill, water-drop size, of medication, it is also made of this number of molecules. There are enough molecules in a drop or pill to supply thousands of molecules to essentially every cell of your brain/body. You could take a bagel and pass it around to thousands of people in a gymnasium. If each person only takes a very small amount it is possible that everyone could get some of the bagel. Yet each of the small amounts could be made of thousands of molecules.

There are about fifty trillion cells in the whole body. Estimates actually range from ten trillion to one hundred trillion. The number is always changing because cells die and new cells are constantly forming. All human beings are also different sizes and shapes and are constantly changing. At any rate, one hundred trillion is 10 to the 14th power. Therefore, when you take a water-drop size pill, about ten thousand parts of the pill could go to each cell in your body/brain.

When you take a pill, the molecules go just about everywhere in your body/brain. However, some parts of your body do not have as much blood supply as other parts and so they do not receive as much of the medication as parts with greater blood supply. There is also a protective physiological mechanism that keeps many chemicals out of the brain. This is called the ***blood/brain barrier***. The walls of the brain ***capillaries***, or very tiny blood vessels, are made of cells that are tightly packed together so that only small molecules can pass through the walls. The capillaries in the brain are also surrounded by a fatty barrier called a ***glial sheath***, or parts of the surrounding ***astrocytes***. These are a certain type of ***glial cell*** that surrounds the neurons. Molecules that are fat soluble are better able to cross the blood/brain barrier.

Chemicals that can cross the blood/brain barrier are called ***psychoactive*** chemicals because they can have effects on the brain.

Chemicals that cannot cross the blood/brain barrier are not psychoactive. Penicillin does not cross the blood/brain barrier and is not good for infections in the brain. It is not psychoactive. Muscle relaxers, opioid pain medications, anticonvulsants, antidepressants, sleeping medications, and anti-anxiety or anxiolytic medications are all psychoactive because they cross the blood/brain barrier. They can affect the brain, make a person groggy, and influence cognition and emotions in many different ways.

100 Billion Neurons

There are about one hundred billion neurons in the whole nervous system. It is difficult to get one's mind around the number one hundred billion. Imagine a professional sports stadium with a capacity for fifty thousand people or so. Imagine that each person in the stadium is a neuron, a single nerve cell in the brain or spinal cord, ready to transmit messages and ready to receive messages from other neurons. The number of neurons in the brain would be equivalent to the number of people in about two million sports stadiums. That would be enough sports stadiums to cover the entire United States, twenty layers thick.

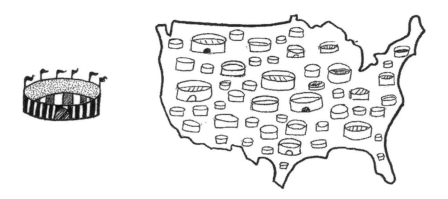

70 percent of all the neurons in the nervous system are in a small area in the back of the brain called the cerebellum. The cerebellum controls coordination. This includes motor coordination, like putting a key into a lock, but also the coordination of thinking, feeling, behaving, and all the other subconscious biochemical processes that occur throughout life's experiences and activities. There are thirty billion neurons or so in the rest of the brain, and about one billion neurons in the spinal cord.

There are about ten to fifty glial cells for each neuron. This comes to about one to five trillion glial cells, which are much smaller than neurons in general and actually take up about the same amount of space as the one hundred billion neurons. These surround the neurons, support them, provide nutrition, and facilitate many other functions.

Each of the billions of neurons has an average of ten to fifteen thousand connections with other neurons. In the cerebellum, many of the billions of neurons have as many as two hundred thousand connections with other neurons. It is said that there are more connections in a single brain than there are stars in the heavens. How would we really know such a thing?

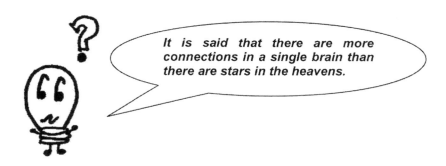

It is said that there are more connections in a single brain than there are stars in the heavens.

Back to the sports stadium analogy. Each neuron or person, with its ten thousand or so connections to other neurons or people, would be able to communicate with ten thousand other neurons or people at once. This would be like sending and receiving messages to ten thousand other people at once. Neurons might tend to talk with others who are close by in the same stadium, but neurons in Minnesota would also be able to talk with neurons in California or Washington or New York all at once.

How does that work?

There are groups of millions of neurons that work together, have the same functions, and send and receive messages to and from other groups of neurons. These groups of neurons that work together are called **nuclei**. There are thousands of brain parts or nuclei, all with specific names, and all working in networks with other nuclei or brain parts.

Each neuron in the group or nuclei receiving its thousands of messages has to decide whether or not to send the messages onto the next neuron. It might be like the game of "telephone" where one person whispers into the ear of another person who then whispers into the ear of the next person in line. Some of the messages received are **excitatory** or "make the neuron more likely to send the message on." Some of the messages are **inhibitory** or "make the neuron less likely to send the message on." There is a part of the neuron called the **axon hillock** which is really responsible for making the final decision whether or not to send the message on down the axon. The axon hillock takes in the thousands of inhibitory and excitatory messages and then makes a decision... send or not send.

Information is sent to other neurons by means of the axon or wire that basically travels away from the cell body toward the next neuron in the line. The next neuron in line receives the information by the **receptors** on the dendrites, on the cell bodies, and even on the axons. These little receiving structures are bundles of proteins formed into specific shapes made ready to receive **neurotransmitters**. Neurotransmitters are chemicals that travel from one neuron to another in order to stimulate the next neuron in line. The receptors might be likened to ears that pick up the sounds and messages from the sending neuron or **pre-synaptic neuron**. The neuron receiving the message is called the **post-synaptic neuron**.

Before the information gets to the axon hillock, it first must travel across the dendrites and the cell body of this pre-synaptic neuron. Information is carried from one side of a particular neuron and then across this neuron to the other side by means of chemical and electrical activity. The information or messages that travel across the specific neuron are like waves of water from a stone thrown into a pond. The wave gets smaller and less strong as it moves across the cell. This is called **decrimation.**

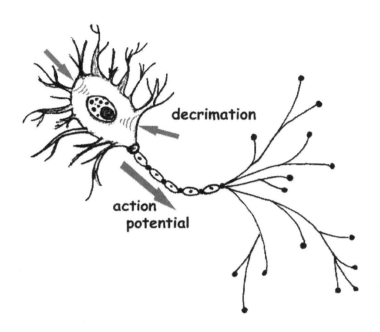

The axon hillock receives these thousands of little wavelets and decides whether or not to send a message down the axon. If it decides to do so, the message traveling down the axon will be extremely strong and clear without any decrimation. This message traveling down the axon is called the **action potential**, and it is an *electrical* message that travels very fast. The message will get to the end of the axon, the axon terminal, and then we have a problem. There is a gap. In general, the neurons do not touch. Instead, there is a space between the neurons. This is called a synapse or a **synaptic gap.** How does the information get across the gap?

Neurotransmitters, Cell Receptors

Information is carried from one neuron to the next by means of chemical messengers, or neurotransmitters, which travel across the synapse. These chemicals squirt out the end of the axon terminals, float across the gap, and influence the next neuron by stimulating its receptors.

There are many neurotransmitters in at least six different categories or types including: acetylcholine, amino acids, monoamines, peptides, purines, and gases. All these neurotransmitters are chemicals that basically stimulate the receptors on the surfaces of each of the billions of neurons. There are millions of receptors on each of the billions of neurons.

Six Main Classes of Neurotransmitters and Subcategories

Acetylcholine

Amino acids
      Glutamate
      GABA
      Aspartate
      (NMDA receptors)
      Others

Monoamines
      Indoleamines
      Catecholamines:
            Dopamine
            Norepinephrine: Sympathetic for postganglionic to effector organs
            Epinephrine

Peptides
      Endorphins
      Substance P
      Neuropeptide Y
      Many others

Purines
      Adenosine
      ATP
      Others

Gases
      Nitric oxide
      Carbon monoxide

Other Chemicals That Influence Transmission

Trophic factors

Hormones
      6 classes of steroid hormones
            estrogens
            androgens
            progestines
            glucocorticoids
            mineralocorticoids
            vitamin D

One might think of the receptors as tiny little baseball gloves all over the surface of the neuron, the dendrites, the cell body, and the axon. These receptor baseball gloves are ready to catch little baseballs, or neurotransmitter chemicals. The baseball gloves can only catch baseballs that fit well in the pocket of the gloves. The gloves have to be open enough to catch the baseballs. The gloves also have to be on the surface and not buried too deeply within the walls or membranes of the neuron.

Neuron

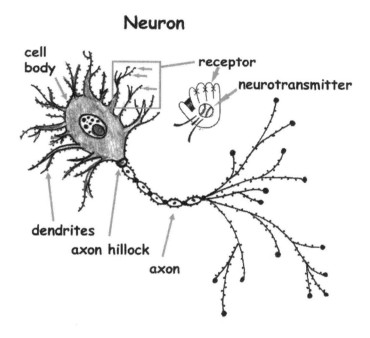

The baseballs, or neurotransmitters, go into the gloves in special and specific ways. They only go into the gloves that are designed to fit them. They are then released or let go by the gloves and go back into the synaptic gap. Then they go back into the gloves and are released again, over and over, even dozens of times per second. This is like "catch and release, catch and release," over and over.

This activity then stimulates the receiving neuron, covered by the gloves or receptors, to experience the message and decide whether or not to send it on down the axon, away from the neuron and on to the next one. As stated earlier, if a chemical makes a neuron more likely to send the message down the axon to the next neuron in line, it is called an excitatory neurotransmitter. If the chemical makes the neuron less likely to send the message on, it is called an inhibitory neurotransmitter. If excitation outweighs inhibition the message will be sent on. If inhibition outweighs excitation the message will not be sent.

Once the receiving gloves have been struck enough by the baseballs, the baseballs are let go completely and are either taken back into the neuron that threw them in the first place (this is called *reuptake* and is like recycling or saving the chemical so it can be used again), or the baseballs are broken down and destroyed by other chemicals in the synapse. This is important to know because mood, anxiety, sleep, and pain are all influenced by the levels of various neurotransmitters floating around between the neurons.

The neurotransmitters do many different things in the brain, spinal cord, nerves, muscles and organs. Various antidepressant medications, antianxiety medications, sleep medications and pain medications all work on neurotransmitters in one way or another. Neurotransmitters are created or manufactured in various neurons, usually in the cell bodies. Then the chemicals themselves are transmitted down the axons of the neurons at a slow transmission speed of one mm per day in the thinnest axons to a fast speed of one hundred mm (3.9 inches) per day in thicker axons. This is a different process than the action potential mentioned above.

The neurotransmitters routinely travel through the blood and cerebrospinal fluid systems as well. When traveling through the blood, they are called *hormones*. Hormones and many other chemicals bathe the neurons (or one might think of the neurons "marinating" in hormones and many other chemicals) which then facilitate either excitatory or inhibitory activity.

The neurons, like all the cells in the body, synthesize or manufacture many chemicals, including neurotransmitters, from precursor molecules derived from the foods we eat. For example, choline in our diet (and from metabolism) plus acetyl-coenzyme A (from metabolism) combine to make acetylcholine. Phenylalanine from our diet can be made by our body into tyrosine, which in turn can be made into dopa, and then into *dopamine*, and then into *norepinephrine*, and then into *epinephrine*. Dopamine, for example, has varied uses in the brain/body. It helps us focus attention. It can help control movement disorders like Parkinson' disease. It is involved in the experiences of pleasure. It helps elevate mood. Epinephrine can elevate mood as well, and can give a sense of increased energy.

L-tryptophan from our diet can be made into 5 hydroxytryptophan which can become *serotonin* (5 hydroxytryptamine, 5HT). However, at this time, there are at least eighteen different kinds of receptors for serotonin in the brain and body, or eighteen different types of baseball gloves that can receive and be stimulated by the serotonin baseball molecules, so to speak. 80–90 percent of the body's serotonin is found in cells in the gastrointestinal tract, but it can also be found in the respiratory tract, in blood vessels, and of course, in the nervous system.

Serotonin will stimulate different receptors in different ways. Serotonin is affected by several antidepressant medications and by many other cognitive and behavioral approaches to depression. Many different antidepressants have different effects on the receptors in different parts of the brain/body. Thus a person may experience relief from depression, but adverse effects such as nausea or dizziness. The person may experience nothing at all or some combination of effects. These effects may be noted at one time in a person's life but may change and result in totally different effects at another time in the person's life.

Serotonin is typically a strong vasoconstrictor of the central and peripheral blood vessels. Associated with some vascular headaches or some types of migraine headaches, platelets may clump in blood vessels and then release serotonin. The serotonin may cause blood vessels in the head to contract or constrict, resulting in less blood flow temporarily and some of the aura or warning symptoms of impending head pain. The increased levels of serotonin may lessen the pain threshold or may increase pain sensitivity or readiness for pain onset. Typically, just before the onset of pain associated with migraines there is an elevated amount of serotonin in the brain. During migraine head pain there is typically a lowered level of serotonin. The lowered amounts may be the cause of the blood vessel dilatation and may account for the throbbing pain experienced during migraine headache.

Of interest is the fact that certain antidepressant medications that increase serotonin, specifically the SSRI's or Selective Serotonin Reuptake Inhibitors including Prozac (fluoxatine), Zoloft (sertraline), Paxil (paroxitine), Lexapro (escitalopram), Celexa (citalopram), etc., can cause vasoconstriction throughout the body. This is what probably accounts for the occasional occurrence of sexual side effects like the lack of libido and lack of ability to reach orgasm at times.

Pain Transmitting Chemicals

It may not be important to know about these various chemicals. However, it is interesting to know that there are many chemicals involved in pain and that pain really is very complicated. We commented already on the chemical serotonin. We tend to think of serotonin as mainly a pain blocking chemical. But it is also a pain transmitting chemical. Serotonin is involved in *inflammation*. Serotonin can cause the blood vessels in the head to contract and can lower the pain threshold, thus contributing to the pain of migraine headaches. Serotonin is also involved in mood difficulties, anxiety, sleep, anger, irritability, and many other emotional and physical experiences.

There are many other chemicals implicated in the transmission of painful messages. These include *Substance P, Histamine, Bradykinin, Prostaglandin, ATP (adenosine tryphosphate), NGF (nerve growth factor) or BDNF (brain derived neurotrophic factor), CGRP (calcitonin gene related peptide), and many others.* If you cut your hand, these chemicals may all be found at the site of injury, but they can also be found in the peripheral nerves transmitting the messages from the site of injury to the spinal cord, the spinal cord itself, and the brain. Some of them, like the NGF (nerve growth factor) or BDNF (brain derived neurotrophic factor), are made in the glial cells of the brain, the cells that support and surround the neurons.

All of these chemicals can irritate pain sensitive nerve endings. This painful stimulation and experience is called *nociception*. *Nociceptors* are sensory nerve endings that receive the noxious or painful messages and begin the reaction to the potentially damaging stimuli by sending nerve signals to the spinal cord and brain. This is different than sensory receptors, nerve endings that receive non-painful messages, like any of the normal sensations of touch, smell, taste, sight, and sound.

Substance P is released from the terminals of specific sensory nerves and used by the nerves to help transmit pain messages from the site of injury into the spinal cord and up to the brain.

Substance P is thought to be significantly elevated in the condition called *fibromyalgia* (more on that later). Substance P is associated with inflammation as well as pain. Inflammation is a complex series of chemical responses in the body that can result in swelling, redness, soreness, and sensitivity to touch. It is part of the body's healing process but can be quite painful.

Substance P is known as a modulator of nociception. It tends to modify the intensity of painful or noxious sensations, typically making them more intense. Substance P is only eleven amino acids long yet it is an integral part of the nervous system involved in pain and psychological stress. Pain is stressful, and stress aggravates pain. Nociceptors themselves, the pain receiving sensory nerve endings, release substance P. This causes *mast cells* to release histamine, which in turn stimulates the nociceptor again. Mast cells are present in many tissues in the body. They are part of the immune system and are typically active in allergies, inflammation, and infection.

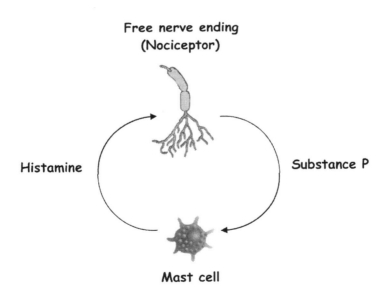

Histamine, another pain transmitting chemical, is found in virtually every cell of the body. It is released by mast cells. It triggers the inflammatory response by facilitating more permeability of capillaries.

This allows more fluid and cell transport across the membranes of the capillaries to fight off infections and foreign invaders. When histamine stimulates nociceptors, it is experienced as an itch rather than pain. We don't know why. We use antihistamines, of course, to relieve the itch. Antihistamines can sometimes lessen pain as well.

Another chemical, bradykinin, is released in the spinal cord in response to nociceptor inputs. It is also released by blood plasma. It acts as a synaptic neuromodulator—changing activity in the synapse. It potentiates or increases ***glutamatergic synaptic transmission.*** This refers to the action of ***glutamate***, the most excitatory neurotransmitter in the brain and spinal cord. It facilitates the action of glutamate which results in more pain hypersensitivity.

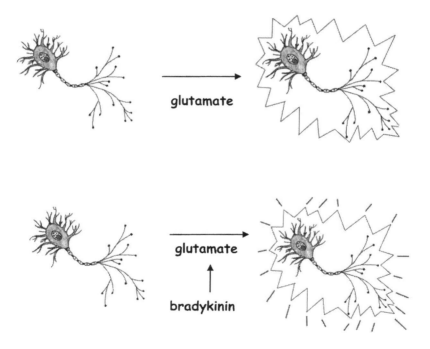

Prostaglandin is another chemical involved in pain transmission. It is involved in many processes in the body and is found and used for different purposes in many organs. One of the purposes is inflammation and fever production. It is released by damaged cells. There is an enzyme called **cyclooxygenase** which helps in the formation or production of prostaglandin. By inhibiting or blocking this enzyme, the synthesis of prostaglandins is blocked, which in turn relieves some of the effects of pain and fever. Celebrex (celecoxib) is a drug that inhibits the action of cyclooxygenase.

Another chemical involved in pain transmission is adenosine triphosphate (ATP). This provides energy and activates capsaicin-sensitive nociceptive **afferent nerves** which are nerves that carry messages from the periphery to or toward the spinal cord and brain. **Capsaisin** is found in hot peppers and is the chemical that draws out substance P from your inner cheeks, tongue, and mouth membranes when you eat the hot peppers. Your own substance P is what causes the hot, painful sensation. If you do this enough, you will deplete your own substance P (only in your mouth, not throughout your body), and the hot peppers will no longer be that hot. Rather, they will just taste good (if you like the taste in the first place) without the significant burn. Repetitive use of capsaicin on an inflamed joint can deplete the substance P in that localized area and temporarily result in less pain.

Nerve growth factor (NGF), or brain derived neurotrophic factor (BDNF), are two more similar chemicals involved in pain transmission. They are pain-related neural modulators that send messages from the periphery to the spinal cord. These chemicals from the periphery and spinal cord, as well as from glial cells, may contribute to the increase in pain during inflammatory **hyperalgesia** which is an increased sensitivity to pain. When a part of the body is red, sore and swollen, it may be hypersensitive to even light touch.

Another chemical involved in pain transmission is calcitonin gene related peptide (CGRP). This is released at the site of injury and results in vaso-relaxation, vaso-dilatation, increased inflammatory responses, and can increase bleeding in the injured area.

Pain Blocking Chemicals

Just as there are many chemicals involved in the process of transmitting painful messages, there are also many chemicals that are intricate in the process of blocking painful messages. The brain doesn't just sit there receiving noxious messages from the body. It also sends messages down the spinal cord to try to block out the pain.

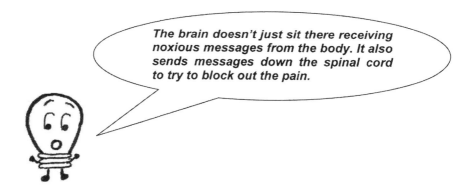

The brain doesn't just sit there receiving noxious messages from the body. It also sends messages down the spinal cord to try to block out the pain.

Some of these chemicals are called *opioid* peptides. You are probably familiar with some of the terms. There are three well-characterized families of opioid peptides produced by the brain/body: *enkephalins* (five amino acids in length), *endorphins* (about sixteen to thirty amino acids in length), and *dynorphins* (similar in length to the endorphins). Endorphins are the most familiar, but all three are a category of pain killing chemicals that the brain/body produces internally. These chemicals are endogenous (made internally by the brain/body) opioid neurotransmitters. Opioid chemicals are like *narcotics* made by your own body. They stimulate the same receptors that opioids or narcotics do, and they are stimulated by and respond to both internal and external opioids and narcotics.

Dopamine is another frequently discussed neurotransmitter. It has many uses in the brain/body. In some parts is helps control smooth and coordinated movements of our limbs and body. In other parts it facilitates focus and attention. In still other parts is helps us to organize our thoughts in logical and orderly patterns. And finally, in some parts of the brain/body it facilitates pleasurable sensations.

Gamma-Amino-Butiric-Acid (GABA), is the most inhibitory neurotransmitter throughout the nervous system. It helps calm hypersensitive and hyperactive nervous system functions such as pain and anxiety. Antiepileptic or antiseizure medications typically make GABA work better. This is why anti-epileptic or anti-seizure medications like gabapentin (neurontin) and others can sometimes help to control pain. They inhibit or calm down electrical nerve transmission.

Two other chemicals involved in blocking pain are serotonin and norepinephrine. There are two main brain areas involved in manufacturing these chemicals to block pain. These are the *raphe magnus nucleus* and the *locus coeruleus*. Serotonin is manufactured in the raphe magnus nucleus and norepinephrine in the locus coeruleus, and both are sent throughout the nervous system and body to help block out pain. The raphe magnus nucleus is in the upper part of the brain stem. The locus coeruleus is a small structure in the pons—the middle of the brain stem. Locus coeruleus means "dark blue place." This structure is fairly inactive most of the time and quite silent during sleep. But it is very active when pain is significant.

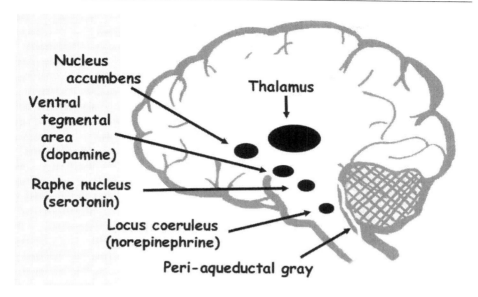

Nucleus accumbens

Ventral tegmental area (dopamine)

Raphe nucleus (serotonin)

Locus coeruleus (norepinephrine)

Thalamus

Peri-aqueductal gray

Other brain and spinal cord parts and networks are involved in blocking out pain. One brain part called the ***peri-aqueductal gray (PAG)*** sends messages, by means of the enkephalins, to the raphe magnus nucleus. In turn, cells from the raphe magnus nucleus send messages, by means of serotonin, down to the dorsal horn of the spinal cord to help block painful messages from traveling up the spinal cord.

There is a lot of activity in the dorsal horn of the spinal cord. Certain neurons in this area of the spinal cord, called the ***lamina II or the substantia gelatinosa***, send out more enkephalins or dynorphins. These then bind to ***mu-opioid receptors*** (stimulating them to block the transmission of painful messages) on A-delta and C fibers. Remember that these fibers are the pain transmitting fibers, or wires, that travel and transmit painful messages from your body, like from a cut on your finger, up your arm into the spinal cord. The *mu*-opioid receptors are proteins consisting of about 370–400 amino acids.

The *mu*-opioid receptors are like the little baseball gloves that have an affinity for a special kind of baseball: the opioids. The opioids, the narcotic pain killers, can be either manufactured in the brain/body or administered from outside the body. Activation of *mu*-opioid receptors inhibits release of substance-P, thus blocking pain to a degree.

The locus coeruleus is activated and gives off or emits impulses in response to meaningful events. When it is stimulated by a stressful or arousing experience such as pain, it releases norepinephrine. This neurotransmitter facilitates and strengthens storage of recent memories and increases wakefulness. It can increase a person's level of energy. It is similar to serotonin in that it stimulates the dorsal horn in such a way to ultimately block the release of substance-P and thus lessen pain.

However, the action of the locus coeruleus can be blocked by opioids. When the locus coeruleus is blocked by opiate drugs or endorphins the result is decreased memory storage and decreased response to stress. Opioid narcotics lessen your ability to remember, and they make you more apathetic to events around you. You may become less motivated to do anything. This is called *avolition*. The following case studies provide further insight into this condition.

Dan, a forty-two-year-old patient who has been on 2500 mg of Morphine per day for about ten years, described his life and daily activity as sitting in front of the television day after day for all those years. He was divorced, but during that ten year period, he had partial custody of his three children. His children would ask him something and he would respond minimally and without enthusiasm. This went on year after year. After he weaned off the opioids over an eight month period, he stated that he had increased motivation and energy. He dated, remarried, and returned to former activities, including riding his motorcycle. His children were older but they started connecting with him again. He was very pleased to be off the medication. He still had pain, but "no worse than before," he stated.

Fred was on opioids at a cost of about $7,500 each month, not counting other medications and office visits. He appeared dull and flat in his presentation and affect, as might be expected. As we discussed his pain situation with him, he answered questions appropriately but very slowly. When we talked with his wife, and didn't pay too much attention to Fred for a minute or so, he would nod off. He was not aware of his own level of cognitive somnolence. He participated in a pain management program and gradually weaned off opioids over several months. Afterward, he described having "less pain." He still had pain, but he was happy, alert, smiling, and enthusiastic.

Linda suffered seven compressed vertebrae in her back associated with severe osteoporosis and trauma. She had a significant and painful peripheral neuropathy due to underlying medical problems. She was also using opioids: Methadone 7.5 mg four times a day and about forty Percocet tablets per month. She had been on this dose of medication for about six years without escalation of use and no misuse. She remained working essentially full time, cared for her daughter and husband, slept normally, exercised every day, and her pain levels were about three on a scale of zero to ten. She was very pleased with this treatment protocol.

Linda's was an unusual situation. Most people would develop tolerance and need more and more of the medication to do the same job. Most would continue to experience higher pain levels in spite of the medication, and maybe even because of the medication to a degree, and would not be able to function as well as Linda. She stated, "People make decisions to drop out of life, not consciously, but they get into a place where they cannot get themselves out of the situation. Movement is the key. If you are not stimulated, you will not be living. A person's identity becomes this 'sick person' rather than 'it does not define me.' This is not who I am." We talked about the idea that people certainly do not choose to be miserable. However, she insisted that there is a level of choice in the whole experience of long-term pain.

One must be very careful with the use of opioids. Opioid use can be a very slippery slope leading to major difficulties. Tolerance, physical dependency, overuse and misuse, and hyperalgesia can all occur. These are not always problems of course, but are probably more common than people realize.

Peripheral Pain Mechanisms

Nerve Endings, Sensory Receptors

We have looked at some of the elements of the nervous system and the brain/body on a microscopic, cellular, biochemical level. Now let's look at the nervous system and the brain/body parts and networks on a larger scale.

There are many different types of sensations associated with touch, temperature, and pain. These are experienced by many varied nerve endings. You can tell the difference between a warm drop of oil and a cold touch of steel. You can tell the difference between a warm breeze and a sharp point. There are nerve endings that are sensitive to these various stimuli essentially everywhere on your body.

There are specialized nerve endings that can sense painful stimuli, called free nerve endings, but there are also many different and specialized nerve endings that sense non-painful messages. There are non-pain sensing nerve endings and receptors for steady skin indentation, vibration, flutter, and itch. Different types of receptors in the skin, muscles, and internal organs are on the receiving, sensing ends of several different types of fibers. This is like many different types, sizes, and shapes of hands on many different types, sizes, and shapes of arms. The varying sensory receptors are waiting and ready to receive messages as they arrive. The receptors that are sensitive to various types of painful stimuli and non-painful stimuli are very important. But the fibers that transmit the messages from the nerve endings to the spinal cord are also extremely important when trying to understand pain. These transmitting wires or fibers will be discussed shortly, but first we will comment briefly on the non-pain sensitive nerve endings.

There are four differently structured nerve endings on the receiving ends of the non-pain transmitting wires. Each can be stimulated alone but are usually stimulated in combination with many other nerve endings at the same time. This is why there can be many different sensations at the same time during any particular experience. The four non-pain sensitive nerve endings include Merkel's cells and Ruffini's corpuscles which are both sensitive to steady skin indentation and tend to adapt slowly to a stimulus. We get used to our clothes on our skin and our glasses on our face but it takes a little time. Pacinian corpuscles are sensitive to vibration and Miessner's corpuscles are sensitive to flutter. Both tend to adapt fairly quickly to a stimulus.

These are the four different nerve endings that are sensitive to non-painful stimuli that have to do with touch. As we all know, there are other nerve endings that have to do with others sensations such as sight, sound, smell and taste. These can be stimulated in unusual ways as well. Pushing on the eyeball might stimulate visual nerve endings and the person might "see stars." Thinking about your favorite food might actually stimulate the taste and smell pathways, or even pathways that have to do with texture or emotions. Just as there are four types of sensory nerve endings that tell us about non-painful touch stimuli, there are other nerve endings that tell us about other stimuli. One of these is the *free nerve endings* that tell us about painful stimuli.

Nociceptors

In the skin and other body organs and tissues there are special sensory nerve endings, free nerve endings called nociceptors, that are sensitive to various painful stimuli. These receptors pick up the information and begin the process of transmitting the information centrally into the spinal cord and then up to the brain.

Pain is detected by free nerve endings exclusively. Some free nerve endings or pain receptors can detect many types of stimuli at the same time. Other free nerve endings are more specialized. There are free nerve endings that detect temperature. Some free nerve endings detect heat and others detect cold. Some heat sensitive free nerve endings do not detect heat when it is too hot, and some free nerve endings do not respond to extremely cold stimuli. You can feel extreme heat and extreme cold but not as hot or cold, only as pain. Also our temperature receptors tend to adapt over time. You get used to the temperature of the hot or cold water, or other stimuli, if it is not too hot or cold to be painful.

Thermal nociceptors pick up painful messages that have to do with temperatures that are too high or low. ***Chemical nociceptors*** respond to external chemicals that can cause tissue damage (acid), and they respond to a variety of internal chemicals released when tissue damage is imminent or has actually occurred (lactic acid). ***Mechanical nociceptors*** respond to pressures that are too strong and can signal impending tissue damage. They also respond to cuts and blows.

There are also ***polymodal receptors*** which can respond to all of the above stimuli. These are receptors that can be stimulated by many different noxious and pain producing stimuli. All these nerve endings are located almost everywhere throughout the body including the skin, bone, connective tissue, muscle, and viscera.

Silent or sleeping nociceptors stay quiet, but can become sensitive to various stimuli when inflammation is involved in the area. When there is tissue damage many chemicals are released into the area of damage. These chemicals are sometimes called an ***inflammatory soup***. This acidic mixture stimulates and sensitizes the various nociceptors into a condition called hyperalgesia. This is the Greek word for "super pain." This is a complex phenomenon that is not well understood.

Transmitting Fibers

In the peripheral nervous system there are different types of specific nerve fibers that transmit messages or information from the stimulated area of the body to the spinal cord. From there, these messages are transmitted up to the brain. The fibers from the periphery to the spinal cord are called *primary afferent fibers*. They are the fibers that first experience the sensory message and begin the process of transmitting it to the spinal cord and then up to the brain. These fibers are specifically named by letters, A, B, C, as well as Greek alphabet letters, for example, A-alpha, A-beta, A-delta and C-nerve fibers.

Messages that are not painful or noxious are transmitted by A-alpha and A-beta fibers. A-alpha fibers carry messages at about 80–120 meters per second or an average of four hundred miles per hour. They typically carry messages that have to do with proprioception or position sense. For example, you know where your feet are without looking. You can touch your nose with your eyes closed.

The A-beta fibers carry messages at speeds of 30–70 meters per second or about two hundred miles per hour. These are the fibers that carry messages about skin indentation, vibration, flutter, light touch, and other non-painful, non-noxious messages.

Messages that are painful, or some messages about temperature, are transmitted by A-delta and C fibers. A-delta messages travel about 5–35 meters per second or about thirty miles per hour. They transmit messages about sharp, pricking pain. C fibers carry messages even more slowly, 0.5–2 meters per second or about one to four miles per hour, and typically about burning pain. These also carry messages about itch.

These primary afferent fibers or axons come in different diameters and are divided into different groups based on their size. The largest diameter fibers are the fastest and the thinnest diameter fibers are the slowest. The thicker the nerve fiber, the faster the information can travel through it. A-alpha, A-beta and A-delta nerve fibers are insulated with myelin. C-nerve fibers are *unmyelinated*.

Myelinated means that the axon of the nerve cell has a surrounding insulating envelope of fatty tissue that facilitates faster transmission of nerve impulses. Unmyelinated means that there is no surrounding insulation and therefore transmission of messages is slower.

Primary Afferent Axons

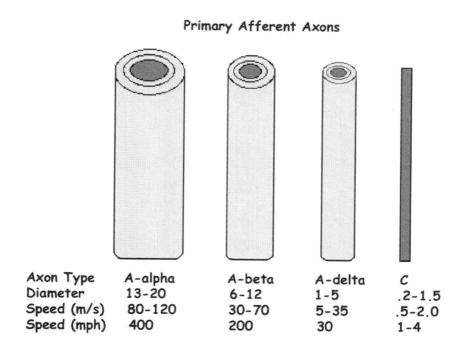

Axon Type	A-alpha	A-beta	A-delta	C
Diameter	13-20	6-12	1-5	.2-1.5
Speed (m/s)	80-120	30-70	5-35	.5-2.0
Speed (mph)	400	200	30	1-4

This sets the foundation for understanding some ideas concerning pathology in the system. It is difficult to understand why pain is experienced sometimes with even very little stimulation or when experiencing sensory stimulation that normally would not be painful. Why does gentle or cold touch hurt sometimes? Why does wind or even slightly rough texture of some clothing hurt an affected skin area? Is there something wrong with the sensory receptors? Is there something wrong with the peripheral primary afferent transmitting fibers? Is there something else going on in the nervous system or the whole brain/body?

David fell off a ladder and injured his knee. Years later the pain in David's knee hurt terribly when the fold of the jeans would rub on the skin. He would wear shorts as much as he could, but in the winter long underwear would prevent some of the rubbing of the jeans.

Paula had four surgeries on her foot. It started out as a simple bunyonectomy, but there were many complications, including infection. After it was finally healed, and for years later, it felt like "a cutting heat" even to touch the skin at all. She would wear Lidoderm patches—a local anesthetic in an adhesive patch—on the foot. This would help, but it hurt terribly when she pulled the patch off.

What biological, pathological process is occurring in these situations? What is making the knee, the foot, or the nervous system hypersensitive?

Nerve endings and peripheral nerves can be damaged or injured. A sun burn is an example of typically short term peripheral tissue injury. A cut in the skin, fracture of a bone, stretch or tear of a ligament, or crush injuries are also examples of typically short-term nerve ending and/or peripheral nerve problems.

Sometimes the problem is long-term or permanent. The underlying localized pathology and injury may not heal back to its normal or pre-injury state. Scar tissue, inflammation, or other pathology of the nerve endings and/or peripheral nerves or other parts of the nervous system may be part of the ongoing cause of pain.

Sensitization of the peripheral nerves can also be part of the problem. The threshold for activation and response to various peripheral stimuli can be very much lowered, meaning that they might be sensitive to and respond to even minimal stimuli. Even a very light touch or wind or cold can be very painful. The peripheral nerves are not only too sensitive but also too active. Peripheral nerves may begin to send messages into the central nervous system absolutely spontaneously with no identifiable stimulation at all, as far as we know, or with very little peripheral stimulation.

> Peripheral nerves may begin to send messages into the central nervous system absolutely spontaneously with no identifiable stimulation at all, as far as we know, or with very little peripheral stimulation.

Peripheral nerves can develop abnormal *ion channels*: pore-forming proteins that help establish and maintain small electrical voltage differences between the inside and the outside of the cells. The ions are the sodium, magnesium, calcium, and other minerals that flow through the pores. Ion channels might not work normally in areas where the nerves have been damaged. Ions are atoms or groups of atoms with an electric charge. Ions flow through ion channels and facilitate flow of electricity across the cell and down the axon. These ion channel proteins help establish and control the electrical changes and activity of the membrane of all living cells. Without these pores or channels, there would be no messages traveling through nerves. Without the appropriate controls in these membrane pores, there will be abnormal electrical activity. This may be part of the problem of pain experienced by damaged peripheral nerves and abnormal ion channels. The damaged ion channel system may result in too much abnormal electrical activity. This may be another reason why anti-convulsant, anti-epileptic medications work. They "stabilize" the membranes of the cell, sort of like recalibrating the ion channels. These include medications like Neurontin (gabapentin), Lyrica (pregabalin), Trileptal (oxcarbazepine), and many others. These types of medications might modulate the ion channels to be less sensitive and less hyperactive.

Demyelinization, or the breakdown of the myelin sheath or insulation around the axons or wires, can result in abnormal electrical activity and pain. Sometimes damaged nerves can also grow abnormally into a bundle called a *neuroma*. This is a little tumor of nerve tissue that can be very sensitive to the slightest stimulus. It is one example of an actual anatomical change that can occur in nerve tissue that has been injured.

Cross talk can develop between damaged nerves and the remaining undamaged nerves. This is called **ephaptic transmission** or **ephapses**. Normally undamaged nerves fibers send the messages up through the nervous system like they are supposed to. Non-painful messages travel up non-pain transmitting A-alpha and A-beta fibers. Painful messages travel up pain transmitting A-delta and C-fibers. However, damaged nerve fibers might send messages incorrectly through their neighbors. Damage to the nerves might result in a normally non-painful A-fiber sensation, such as light touch, being transmitted to and through a painful C-fiber pathway. This is like a traffic detour when driving. The normally non-painful light touch message gets detoured from the normally non-pain A-fiber road to a C-fiber pain road. Thus, a normally non-painful message, such as a light touch, can hurt. These ephapses, or abnormally connected neuronal fibers, have been found in the peripheral nervous system, the central nervous system, and the autonomic nervous system.

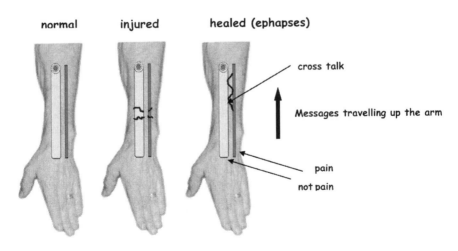

Neurogenic inflammation is swelling or edema of nerves and surrounding tissues. This happens particularly in the peripheral nervous system but also in the central nervous system and/or in the autonomic nervous system. This may be a cause of hypersensitivity and hyperalgesia. Inflammatory neuropeptides, such as Substance P, and others not yet identified, may be released from primary afferent nociceptors and result in spreading of the painful sensation over a larger area of involvement. Prostaglandins may be released from sympathetic post-ganglionic neurons and result in the same type of spreading or enlarging of the painful site. Topical compounded medications using NSAIDs (non-steroidal anti-inflammatory drugs), lidocaine, capsaisin, and others, may work by lessening the inflammation and spreading effects of this type of peripheral, central, and autonomic neuropathic pain.

The ***nervi-nervorum*** is a nerve sheath or membrane around various nerves which has its own nerve supply for sensation. It can be sensitive to pressure, such as from another structure that is not supposed to be there, like a tumor, cyst, blood clot, bullet. It can also be sensitive and compressed by a structure such as a herniated disc in the back or neck that presses on the nerves directly. It should be noted that disc pathology in the neck and back can also result in chemical irritation of nerves. The disc may leak certain chemicals that irritate the surrounding nerves. It may not be only mechanical-pressure-compression causing pain, but also chemical irritation. This, of course, does not show on standard testing. The nervi-nervorum painful stimulation can be lessened by membrane stabilizing medications like anti-epileptic medications and by anti-inflammatory medications.

Central Pain Mechanisms

Spinal Cord Transmission Up To The Brain

Elizabeth, a thirty-seven year old woman with fourteen years of fibromyalgia, stated that she was sure the problem was due to an imbalance in her brain chemistry. She said, "It is the way my brain receives and interprets things. My brain is wired differently." Indeed, things can be wired differently than the usual person. Much of the information the brain receives and interprets comes from the body via the spinal cord. Some of the information comes from the sense organs and enters the brain more directly. Elizabeth could walk into a restaurant and suddenly get a headache due to the very slight smell of cigarette smoke. She could sense even slight mold in a building or carpet and become sickened as a result.

When we feel or experience something unusual or when a person experiences pain for a long time, we might wonder about the wiring of the nervous system. There are many things that can happen throughout the nervous system due to the experience of painful stimuli over time. At this juncture we consider what can happen in the spinal cord as it sends information up to the brain.

The central nervous system (CNS) is that part of the nervous system housed by bone: the spinal cord housed by the vertebral column, and the brain housed by the skull. A nerve tract in the spinal cord that carries messages up to the brain is called the *spinothalamic tract.* This means messages go from the spine to the thalamus. Most sensory messages, pain or otherwise, go to the thalamus, and are then distributed to many other brain parts, centers, and pathways. Many go to the *reticular activating system* where they have significant effects on alertness and sleep. Many go to parts of the *limbic system*. A part of the limbic system called the *anterior cingulate cortex* is where some of the emotional components of the painful experience begin. Messages go to the *amygdala*, another part of the limbic system, where the emotional experiences associated with pain are felt and remembered.

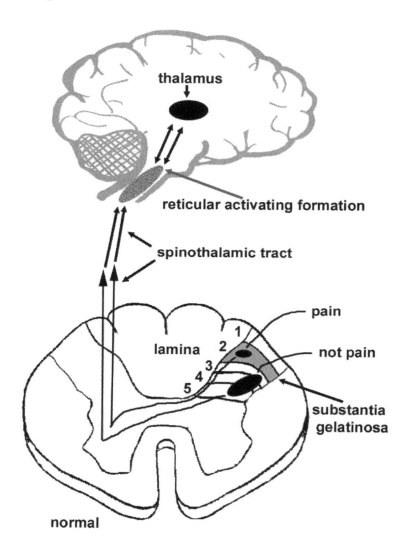

When bombarded by long-term pain, the nervous system responds. Some of the actual wires and cells of the CNS change over time and these changes can persist long after the original pain problem is healed. Normally, adaptive changes of the various parts of the nervous system are referred to as ***plasticity, or neuroplasticity,*** and are thought of as a good thing. Neuroplasticity is the life-long ability of the nervous system networks and pathways to adapt, change, and reorganize based on new experiences.

The nervous system can change and adapt to damage. Certain parts of the nervous system can substitute for other parts that have been damaged, at least to a degree. There is a lot of redundancy and overcapacity in the nervous system. Part of the brain can be damaged and still heal and change, and other parts of the brain might actually take over some of the missing or damaged functions.

However, sometimes the changes that occur are not so helpful or useful. Sometimes the changes can result in pain. Previously we described the fact that normally, painful inputs from the A-delta (thinly myelinated, pain transmitting fibers) and C fibers (small, unmyelinated pain transmitting fibers) go into the dorsal horn of the spinal cord and penetrate to the layer of lamina 1 or 2. The lamina 1 or 2 neurons then transmit the high intensity, noxious, painful signals up the spinal cord to the brain. Normally, the fibers that carry the non-painful messages from the periphery (the A-beta or large myelinated fibers) go deeper into the layers of the spinal cord dorsal horn, lamina 3–5. Then these non-painful messages travel up to the brain.

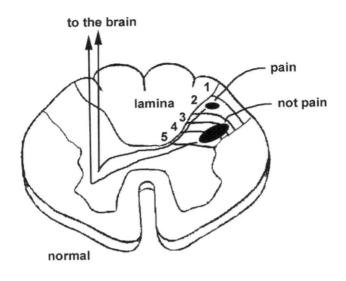

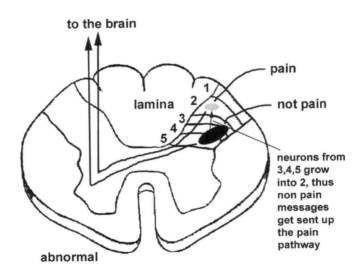

However, after long-term peripheral nerve stimulation involving painful messages, some neurons and their fibers in lamina 1 and 2 can actually die. Fibers from the neurons in deeper lamina

3–5 grow back into lamina 1 and 2 in order to take the place of the cells and fibers that have been excited to death by the long-term painful stimulus. Then normally non-painful messages travel up the spinal cord in the path coming from lamina 1–2, the path that normally carries painful messages. The brain then experiences light touch in the periphery as a painful message coming up the wrong path of the spinal cord. This, indeed, might be one explanation for the abnormal experience or sensation of allodynia, a hypersensitivity to minimal sensation.

Also, some of the nerves of the spinal cord start to send signals up to the brain spontaneously, without input from the periphery. Things can hurt worse for no reason. Sometimes the nerves become very sensitive and seem to respond to very minimal stimuli. Sometimes they send painful messages without any stimulation whatsoever, as far as we can tell.

Also, studies show that an increase in substance P and other pain transmitting chemicals in the central nervous system, the brain, and the spinal cord can result from long-term noxious inputs from the periphery. This can result in a decrease in the opioid binding sites, a *down-regulation* of the opioid receptors, and thus fewer of the normal pain blocking mechanisms by the brain and spinal cord.

Normally, chemicals come out the axon terminals and go across the synapse to stimulate receptor sites on the post-synaptic neuron. There are some chemicals called *retrograde neurotransmitters* that come out of the post-synaptic neuron and go back to the pre-synaptic neuron and stimulate the neuron to excrete more neurotransmitters. Sometimes, in long-term painful states, these retrograde neurotransmitters are overactive and don't let the neurons rest. The neurons keep transmitting messages without need or advantage, and this can be part of the reason for ongoing pain.

Autonomic (Sympathetic) Mechanisms:

Jessica was hit in the face by a PVC pipe that fell several stories from the roof of a building. Years later, even a very light touch on the cheek was like "hot, stabbing fire." In fact, even just approaching Jessica to touch her cheek would make her flinch, grimace, and quickly pull away. Her heart rate increases and she sweats. She said, "It makes me feel like I want to lash out, like an animal might when in pain or trapped. This is frightening to me. I don't understand it. Why does my body act this way? Why do I act this way?"

What biological, pathological process or condition is creating these symptoms? Something is making the sensory nervous system hypersensitive, and her body is responding in very uncomfortable and frightening ways.

The autonomic nervous system is often described as part of the peripheral nervous system. In reality it is mixed in with the central and peripheral nervous systems in intimate and interesting ways. The autonomic nervous system does things automatically. When the lights are turned off in the room your pupils will dilate automatically. This is an autonomic nervous system function. When the lights are too bright the pupils will constrict. Blood pressure, pulse rate, sweating, muscle tone are all controlled automatically, by the autonomic nervous system.

The autonomic nervous system is made of the two parts that work with each other in a balanced choreographic dance. The two parts are the sympathetic nervous system (activated in stressful situations) and the parasympathetic nervous system (much more calm and vegetative). The sympathetic nervous system can be excited by anxiety, anger, depression and pain.

Jessica feels tremendous and instantaneous anxiety when someone approaches her face. Anxiety can stimulate C-fibers in the peripheral nervous system and also the painful message centers in the dorsal horn of the spinal cord. Anxiety and other sympathetically controlled experiences and feelings can worsen pain. This may be part of the mechanism called *sympathetically maintained pain* or *sympathetically mediated pain*. When the sympathetic nervous system is excited, pain can be worsened due to ephaptic messages between peripheral and central sensory and sympathetic fibers. Ephaptic messages, or ephapses, have been found between sensory and sympathetic fibers throughout the nervous system.

Wind-Up

Sensitivity to certain things in life is normal. Normally you may have a favorite smell, you may have a favorite song, and you may or may not know the specific moment or experience from which this came. You have become sensitive to a stimulus, more so than others who do not have that same favorite smell or song.

> Normally you may have a favorite smell, you may have a favorite song, and you may or may not know the specific moment or experience from which this came.

Normally light touch does not hurt. If there is something wrong with the nervous system, light touch might hurt. Depending on what is wrong with the nervous system, other normally non-painful sensations may also hurt. During migraine headaches lights can hurt the eyes and sounds can hurt the ears. Certain conditions might make one too sensitive to smells. Certain conditions can make a person overly sensitive and responsive to emotional situations as well.

Allodynia, a hypersensitivity to minimal stimulation, can also present as a painful sensation and response to a normally non-painful stimulus. Light touch or wind on the skin can hurt. Sheets on the skin of the feet can hurt. These examples are called *mechanical allodynia,* and might be similar to the pain one might feel with a light touch on severely sunburned skin. Interestingly, mechanical allodynia of neuropathic pain may be modulated by anterior cingulate cortex electrical stimulation. Research on rats has demonstrated this. Stimulation of the anterior cingulate cortex has lessened the pain responses associated with mechanical allodynia.

Previously we described the fact that painful neural messages can stimulate free nerve endings wherever they are located in the body. Then these messages are transmitted by specialized A-delta and C fibers from the point of stimulation to the dorsolateral part of the spinal cord. This is where the peripheral nerve wires enter the spinal cord and the messages from the periphery continue their journey up to the brain. This is the normal path of pain stimulation and perception. There is a painful stimulus; the message travels through the nervous system to the brain; the brain/body responds.

Sometimes neurons fire spontaneously or are hyperactive all on their own without any observable stimulus. This can occur at the nerve endings like the fingertip or other parts of the skin. But it can actually occur in any other part of the nervous system including the transmitting fibers and wires up the arm or limb, the pain transmitting mechanisms and wires or tracts up the spinal cord, and the pain and suffering networks in the brain itself.

There are times when the nervous system can act as though there is a particular or specific stimulus, but in reality, there might be none. Or there may indeed be a stimulus but we might not be able to detect or recognize it. In such situations it seems that parts of the nervous system fire for no particular reason or at least none that we can pinpoint.

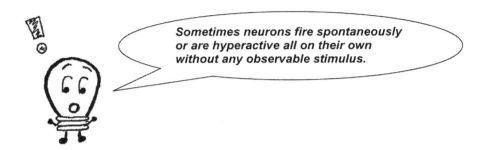

Sometimes neurons fire spontaneously or are hyperactive all on their own without any observable stimulus.

There can be a momentary or ongoing painful experience anywhere in the nervous system without any particular identifiable painful stimulus. This may be hard to believe and is certainly hard to understand, but it is true. This could be part of the problem of long-term pain and normal tests. The nervous system may have developed these repetitively trained pathways of painful experience that now fire even on their own, without specific stimulation.

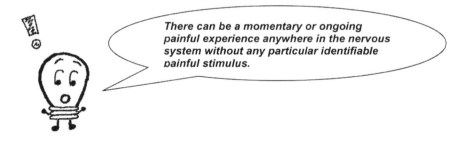

There can be a momentary or ongoing painful experience anywhere in the nervous system without any particular identifiable painful stimulus.

Prolonged repetitive firing of some nociceptor nerve endings, free nerve endings, and their fibers can cause excess release of ***glutamate*** at synapses in the spinal cord. Glutamate, the brain/body's most excitatory and abundant neurotransmitter, acts on ***N-methyl-D-aspartate (NMDA) receptors*** in the spinal cord.

NMDA activation can increase the spinal cord post-synaptic cells' responsiveness to painful stimuli. The activation of NMDA receptors in the spinal cord can also cause the post-synaptic neurons to be more reactive to all types of inputs. This is called a ***central sensitization***. The post-synaptic spinal cord neurons become hypersensitive to all types of inputs, not just painful inputs. Once this happens, the neurons and pathways in the spinal cord can tend to spontaneously fire even without inputs that we can identify.

NMDA antagonists are chemicals that can lessen pain to a degree. These are chemicals that impede the glutamate reception and function, and thus can suppress the experience of pain in animals. One of these chemicals is dextromethorphan. There is some evidence that administration of dextromethorphan with opioids can help prevent central sensitization and can lessen opioid tolerance, at least to a degree.

Normally, it typically does not require much stimulation for us to feel a sensation. Light touch, warmth, and cold can be minimal and still felt and experienced. It often requires more intense stimulation of the various receptors in the body to activate the pain sensitive fibers that carry the messages into the spinal cord and up to the brain. For example, a little heat might simply feel warm and comfortable, whereas too much heat can feel burning and painful. Sometimes the heat, if applied slowly, might take a while to feel uncomfortable. If a frog is dipped in very hot water, it will withdraw its legs quickly and try to escape. However, if the frog is swimming in room temperature water, and the water is heated up gradually, the frog will not try to escape until it is too late.

The pain sensitive nerve endings actually have thresholds of stimulation and activity that need to be reached and surpassed in order for the painful message to be transmitted. Inputs have to be strong enough to actually stimulate the free nerve endings to carry the painful messages along the pain transmitting fibers to the spinal cord and up to the brain. If heat or cold or touch or pressure is strong enough to be painful, and if this input is repetitive, there can be a progressive buildup of the painful experience. Some of this buildup actually occurs in the dorsolateral column of the spinal cord.

Repetitive stimulation of the peripheral nerve with the intensity sufficient to activate the pain sensitive fibers leads to a progressive buildup of the magnitude of electrical response in the spinal cord. Thus, repeated strong messages from the peripheral nerves buildup the electrical responses in the spinal cord. It takes less and less stimulus to bring about the pain transmitting response in the spinal cord.

Repetitive stimulation of the peripheral nerve with the intensity sufficient to activate the pain sensitive fibers leads to a progressive buildup of the magnitude of electrical response in the spinal cord.

This is like priming the pump on a motor. When you repetitively pump the primer bulb on the lawn mower to force gas into the engine, the mower becomes more ready to respond and start when you pull the starter cord. In the nervous system this is referred to as *wind-up*. The spinal cord becomes more sensitive and more ready to receive messages from the periphery and send them up to the brain. Once the motor or pump is primed, it doesn't require as much work or stimulation to send the message all the way up to the brain. Now the person may experience pain when the stimulus is minimal or even negligible. The anatomy and biochemistry of the spinal cord has been changed.

> *Once the motor or pump is primed, it doesn't require as much work or stimulation to send the message all the way up to the brain.*

In more complex terms, it can be stated that persistent stimulation of peripheral nerves can lead to disproportionate up-regulation of the central nervous system or the spinal cord and brain. The central nervous system becomes more sensitive and responds in a maladaptive manner. This persistent pain can be associated with three specific clinical phenomena. These are *hyperalgesia, hyperpathia, and allodynia.*

Hyperalgesia means that there is an increased response to a painful stimulus. If you are stuck in the finger by a pin, and you rate the pain as a three out of ten, this might be described as your baseline response to this painful stimulus. The sensory nerve endings in the finger, the transmitting wires and fibers from these nerve endings up the arm to the spinal cord, the spinal cord pathways that send the messages up to the brain, and the brain itself are all involved in this experience. If there is something wrong with this system, such as that the person feels a standard pinprick sensation as a nine out of ten, this is called hyperalgesia.

Again, the receptors in the spinal cord that receive the painful messages from the periphery are called NMDA receptors. It is possible to a degree to block these receptors from receiving the painful messages. Various medications work in this way, but may not work very well. These include, but are not limited to, opioids and anti-epileptic drugs, which not only have effects on the brain and spinal cord, but may also have effects on the peripheral nerves and autonomic systems. Research is constantly being done to find other chemicals and medications and ways to block painful messages.

Research is also being done to try to further understand hypersensitivity and hyperreactivity phenomena. Some very interesting things have been discovered in the spinal cord associated with long-term painful inputs. We described one of these phenomena earlier. Remember those thinly myelinated A-delta fibers that transmit painful messages penetrate to the layer of lamina 1 and 2 of the dorsolateral part of the spinal cord? Unmyelinated C-fibers, also pain transmitting fibers, penetrate to lamina 2 as well. Sometimes repetitive stimulation of the pain transmitting nerves and the long-term experience of pain results in an atrophy or dying off of some of the C fiber nerve endings just after they enter the spinal cord. As stated earlier, the body seems to compensate by filling in the open nerve fiber areas with the A-beta fibers which are non-pain message transmitting fibers. Thus, normally non-noxious stimuli begin to hurt or send painful messages up the spinal cord so that the brain thinks that the stimulus is a painful one.

Interestingly, and for unknown reasons, the A-beta non-pain transmitting fibers begin to secrete or use the pain transmitting neurotransmitter Substance P in this process as well. Normally the non-painful message transmission system does not use Substance P in the non-pain message transmission process. But the normally non-painful message transmitted by A-beta fibers, by using substance P, becomes a painful message. Light touch hurts. Sound and light can hurt during migraine headache. Wind or cold or warmth or sheets or clothes can hurt on very sensitive skin areas. The person may become very sensitive, uncomfortably so, to many stimuli that normally would not be uncomfortable. If one could change the A-beta fibers back to normal, or prevent the C-fibers from dying off in the spinal cord, or prevent the A-beta fibers from secreting substance P, or block the pain transmission capabilities, maybe the painful experience could be changed significantly.

Allodynia, described earlier, is a painful sensation and response to a normally non-painful stimulus. Hyperpathia is similar to allodynia. Once the stimulation or light touch is discontinued, there may be a residual ongoing painful experience and response. This ongoing sensation, after the stimulus has stopped, may be painful or not, depending on the stimulation and the nervous system. A patient described hyperpathia by stating, "When I am poked it hurts, but after it is released, the pain still grows for a while."

Imagine that you are a neuron or some other part of the nervous system. Imagine that you are alone in the dark and afraid of the dark. In this situation you might be hypersensitive and hyperresponsive to sounds. Even the slightest sounds can make you jump. You might even jump when there is no sound at all but somehow you think there is a sound. This is similar to the hypersensitivity and hyperreactivity of the nervous system when it has been bombarded by painful messages for a long time or when associated with significant stress during that time. The following case examples are illustrative of these phenomena.

Mary, a thirty-five-year-old woman with fibromyalgia, osteoarthritis, anxiety with panic attacks, sleep apnea, and nicotine dependency, has been using about two Percocet per day for several years. She is also very creative, artistic, has a great sense of humor, is supportive to her family, and has a fairly good relationship with her husband. She wonders why her pain is worse when she is feeling more anxiety. She states, "Sometimes a light touch on my skin can feel like a bee sting, and it continues after the person has stopped touching me. Goosebumps form when something is very interesting to me."

These are examples of allodynia (light touch hurts), hyperpathia (it keeps hurting after the touching stops), and sympathetic hypersensitivity and hyperreactivity (goosebumps). But pain is even more complicated. It is affected by the stress of perceived injustice and lack of sense of control.

Brad, a thirty-five year old construction worker, hurt his back while lifting. He went through spinal fusion surgery and revision two times within the first two years after the injury. He then underwent a nerve root injection in the left S1 region which did not help, but instead left him with significant pain in the leg. As part of his treatment he tried a spinal cord stimulator which worked somewhat at first, but later stopped working and was eventually taken out. He was treated with high dose opioids off and on for several years. He used Methadone, Duragesic and Vicodin in *equianalgesic* (see glossary for conversion table comparing opioid strengths) doses of about 30-40 Vicodin or Percocet tablets per day. He weaned down on the medications but remained on about 6 per day. He stated, "Behind my left leg, in the thigh, it feels like it is frozen solid and someone is rubbing on it really hard. My left foot feels like it is throbbing when there is any pressure on it at all; I mean, even my sock. When I get home I will take off my sock. I wear really loose shoes. I put on shorts at home so that there will be minimal touching of the skin. I try not to sit on my left buttock or thigh at all. Even in the car I slip off my left shoe. I wear the shorts in the winter even, even when I go shopping at the Mall of America." As time went by he actually became more stable with respect to his medication use and began to work full time. Pain bothered him less after he settled his case with the insurance carrier and felt much less stress.

Neuropathic pain might also be associated with genetics and early environmental upbringing and experience. Kathy, a forty year old woman with fibromyalgia, asked if her condition was related to hypersensitivity to things when she was very young. She stated that when she was very young she was like the girl in *Hans Christian Anderson's story The Princess and the Pea. She stated that her pain seemed weird, complex, misunderstood, and to her the intensely sensitive experience of pain was similar to the experience of the princess. The princess could feel the pea under many layers of mattresses. Kathy could feel pain with very little stimulation.*

Jennifer, who also struggled with fibromyalgia, remembered that when she was young she had to have the bows on her shoes in the exact place. She remembered having to cut the tags out of her shirts. She thought about how the inside pocket of her jeans bothered her leg when sitting down. She recalled that the wrinkles in sheets were irritating. She wondered if fibromyalgia could be spotted in early childhood or if it could be predicted. As far as we know, there is no clear correlation between hypersensitivity in childhood and the development of fibromyalgia in adulthood. But it is an interesting question.

Laura described her pain by stating, "It feels like someone is beating on my head. It feels like a rope is pulling from my feet to my head. All my nerves are overactive, like after helping someone move all their furniture from an apartment to a house. That is how I feel all the time. If one thing affects someone in one way, I seem to be affected ten times worse. My body has turned against me."

These people experience hypersensitivity in various parts and networks of their nervous systems. Their nervous systems are hypersensitive and hyperreactive. Some people experience nociceptive pain, but others have neuropathic pain or something wrong with the pain sensing and responding systems. Many people have both.

Nociceptive Vs. Neuropathic Pain

Nociceptive

←——————————————————→

Neuropathic

The nervous system is working and doing what it is supposed to do.

The nervous system is damaged, changed, and not working correctly.

Nociceptive pain is typically protective pain. In nociceptive pain the nervous system is functioning normally. It sounds the alarm concerning possible tissue damage. The nerves are working. They are doing what they are supposed to do. They are not damaged.

Nociceptive pain can be categorized as either **somatic** or **visceral**. Somatic pain is more localized in the peripheral body, like when you hit your thumb with a hammer; it is more constant, sharp, defined, specific, aching, and/or throbbing. Visceral is in the abdominal or internal organs of the body, like a stomach ache; it is more diffuse, vague, generalized, off and on, and colicky.

Nociceptive pain can occur due to chemical stimulation such as when exposed to acid, or thermal pathology such as a burn, or mechanical stimulation such as a cut. Pain can be nociceptive or **neuropathic,** or a combination of both. Neuropathic pain, caused by damage to the nervous system itself, is often described as burning, tingling, shooting, cold, hot, pins and needles, like asleep and extremely painful all the time, or most of the time. Neuropathic pain can be the result of pathological changes in any of the parts of the nervous system, the peripheral nervous system, the central nervous system, the autonomic nervous system, and the interactions between the systems. There can be allodynia, hyperpathia, and hyperalgesia. The damage can be associated with hypersensitization of the parts of the nervous system or networks, or damage to the inhibitory functions (that would normally calm down painful messages) of some of the nervous system networks.

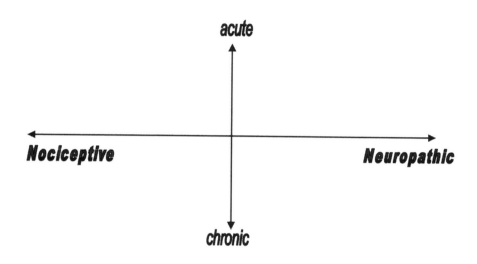

Pain can also be acute or chronic. Pain can come on quickly and last a short time. You sprained your ankle yesterday. This is "acute pain." You sprained your ankle a few weeks ago and it still hurts. This is called "subacute pain." This may simply be a matter of semantics with respect to the duration of a painful experience, but in acute and subacute situations the concept "if it hurts, don't do it" probably applies.

"Chronic" means that the pain lasts a long time, beyond the healing phase, is not really protective, and does not really get better with time and rest. It may have lost its protective purpose. It is not telling you to see the doctor and find out what is wrong. You already did that. It is not telling you to give it time to heal. You already did that. It is not telling you to rest it. You already did that. In fact, you continue to rest it without real benefit, and you probably experience significant worsening of the effects of pain in your life. The more you rest, the harder it is to get up and do things. The harder it is to get up and do things, the more you rest. These terms, acute, subacute, and chronic are fairly arbitrary definitions. All of them can be nociceptive and/or neuropathic.

Pain mandates responses from us, and sometimes we acquiesce with brain/body activities, thoughts, feelings, and behaviors that are not really helpful. The brain experiences the pain. The brain responds and initiates many actions in the brain/body.

Pain mandates responses from us, and sometimes we acquiesce with brain/body activities, thoughts, feelings, and behaviors that are not really helpful.

PART 2

BEYOND THE BASICS

Triune Brain

Paul D. MacLean (May 1, 1913 – December 26, 2007) was an American physician and neuroscientist who made significant contributions in the fields of physiology, psychiatry, and brain research through his work at Yale Medical School and the National Institute of Mental Health. MacLean proposed that the human brain was in reality three brains in one: the **reptilian complex**, the **limbic system**, and the **neocortex**. This has been described as the "evolutionary triune brain theory."

Triune Brain

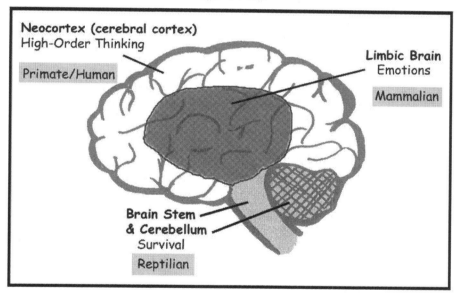

The "reptilian brain" includes the brain stem and cerebellum. The term reptilian brain comes from the fact that a reptile's brain is dominated by the brain stem and cerebellum which control instinctive survival behavior. These brain parts control the muscles, balance and coordination, and many autonomic functions or things that occur automatically. This includes temperature, pulse, breathing, blood vessel dilatation and constriction, dilatation and constriction of pupils, sweating, blushing, goose flesh. This brain system is quickly responsive to acute and immediate changes and stresses in the environment, both external and internal, including pain.

MacLean first introduced the term limbic system in a paper in 1952. This has been referred to as "the old mammalian brain." The limbic system is the source of emotions and instincts, like feeding, fighting, fleeing, and sexual behavior. Stimulation of this part of the brain, naturally or experimentally by mild electric current, produces emotions. This is an extremely important part of the brain when trying to understand pain and suffering.

The surface of the brain is active when we are thinking as human beings, not just reacting or functioning as other animals or higher order mammals. This is also called the neocortex or the ***cerebral cortex***. It is similar to the brain of higher mammals, but unique to humans as it controls even higher-order thinking skills such as reasoning, speech, and salience or self-awareness. It helps us to fill out our tax forms, write symphonies, and plan for our children's educations.

The deeper brain parts, the limbic system and the reptilian system, function on a more instinctual level, subconscious level. The neocortex and its higher order functioning is uniquely human. However, there are impressive examples of animal behaviors that we do not fully understand. Nor do we understand the inner world of animals such as their problem solving abilities, language and communication, empathy and possibly altruism.

In human beings, all of these brain parts and networks are involved when a person is experiencing pain and suffering. Problems can occur in all these brain areas which can either aggravate or ameliorate pain. Thoughts can change pain. Emotions can change pain. Subconscious autonomic nervous system activity can change pain. Behaviors can change pain. Human beings can modify and control their thoughts, feelings, behaviors, and subconscious autonomic functions at least to a degree.

Learning, Long-Term Potentiation (LTP)

The entire brain, and for that matter, all the parts of the nervous system and brain/body, are involved in learning, remembering, responding, experiencing and repeating. Learning at the microscopic, cellular, biochemical level might account for much of the painful experiences, flare-ups, usual responses, and even self-defeating behaviors. Learning something new and changing responses can account for relief and rehabilitation as well.

Long-term potentiation (LTP) is the cellular, microscopic, biochemical, synaptic model for learning of thoughts, feelings and behaviors. It involves the process of stimulating the receptors on the dendrites over and over, until eventually it doesn't require much stimulus to bring about the response. A dense cluster of rapid action potentials will facilitate long-term potentiation. Practicing something over and over helps us to learn long-term. Repetitive pumping of the primer bulb on the lawn mower makes it easier to start the mower. It requires less stimulus, pulling the starter cord once or twice, to bring about the response, starting the mower. At the neuron level the synapses become hypersensitive and hyperresponsive to various stimuli. The synapses become primed, warmed up, ready for action at the slightest stimulus. After potentiation has occurred the pathway is stronger. There is an increased likelihood that a single or simple stimulus will result in an action potential, or the transmission of the message down the axon.

All persons are born with genetic traits similar to all other humans, but each person has very specific and unique individual traits. Each person is raised in an environment which may be similar to others or may be quite unique to the individual. Each person learns many things similar to others but again unique and specific to the individual. We may have practiced certain behaviors in the past, or are presently practicing certain behaviors, that are helpful or hurtful. We may be practicing behaviors that can actually cause or contribute to the problems we are currently experiencing. The genetic traits we have been given and what we practice over time are the foundations of learning.

There are usually many components of learned thought, feelings and behaviors associated with medical conditions that impact the nervous system. As we learn to understand this, we may also learn to understand things we can do to make healthy changes, things that can actually lessen pain, or things that can help one to live better with what remains.

Let's describe learning and memory on a cellular level. This really involves the strengthening of connections between neurons. It normally requires a certain amount of stimulation for a message to be sent from one neuron to the next. A pin prick is a stimulus and the message travels from one neuron to the next and up into the brain because of this particular amount and type of stimulation. When connections between neurons are strengthened it means that it requires less stimulation for a particular message to be sent from one neuron to the next. There are three main phenomena that we will address. These are *specificity, cooperativity,* and *associativity.*

Specificity refers to the specific active synapses and the results of repetitive active stimulation at these synapses. If some of the synapses onto a cell have been highly active, and others have not been active, only the active ones become strengthened. If you practice a measure of piano music over and over in a particular or specific way, then this is what you will learn. If you experience pain and practice only specific thoughts, feelings, behaviors, then this will become your expertise.

Cooperativity refers to simultaneous stimulation by two or more axons at the same time, pairing. Nearly simultaneous stimulation by two or more axons produces LTP much more strongly than repeated stimulation by just one axon. Imagine you are practicing a particular piece of music on the piano when all of a sudden an earthquake shakes the neighborhood. These two events may become paired or conjoined in memory forever. From then on, every time you hear that music you feel the fear of the earthquake experience. Or if you are exposed to an earthquake again, you may hear that song in your head. Then later, if you are exposed to any similar stressful situation, you may hear that song in your head. These pairings become "hardwired," strong, and difficult to change.

As a result of specificity and cooperativity there are certain changes in the nervous system that can account for some of the perpetually strong and hypersensitized painful experiences. Imagine axons and synapses are activated throughout the nervous system when pain and anger are paired together. Imagine that whenever there is pain, there is also a sense of anger or frustration or lack of control. These pairings become very strong and hard to change. Other things might be paired with pain, such as taking pills and resting. Many things are often repeatedly activated together and thus become hard to separate.

In general, do anger and a sense of lack of control make pain better or worse? Imagine that axons and synapses throughout the nervous system that are related to joy and gentle activity are essentially inactive. Imagine that this is the case even while the axons and synapses related to the pain and anger pathways and networks are very active. The synapses of pain and anger pathways and networks become strengthened. The synapses of joy and gentle activity pathways and networks remain the same or weaken. *Neurons that fire together wire together. Neurons that don't fire together don't wire together.*

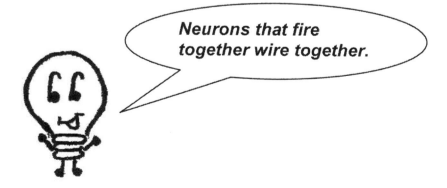

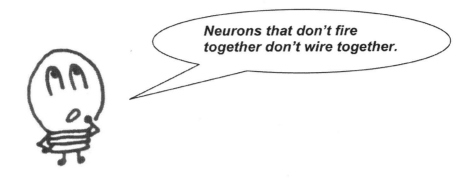

Neurons that don't fire together don't wire together.

Associativity refers to pairing a weak input with a strong input. A person experiences the pain of accidentally cutting off his fingers with a circle saw. The saw was dull and started to catch and burn the wood of the board it was cutting. The smell of slightly burning wood, or the sound of a saw, might be the weak input. The pain of the injury might be the strong input. Associativity refers to pairing that will enhance later responses to the weak input. The person might feel pain or anxiety when simply smelling burning wood or hearing a circle saw.

Relatively weak stimuli or triggers can result in significant or severe flare-ups of pain. Just the thought or sight of the place of injury can stimulate a flare-up of pain. Is it possible that relatively weak comfort triggers or experiences could result in significant calming or lessening of the painful experience?

There are actual anatomical, biochemical changes that occur in the nervous system when we learn something. When we are learning, the whole transmission of messages from neuron to neuron is **up-regulated**. This involves at least four basic biological processes.

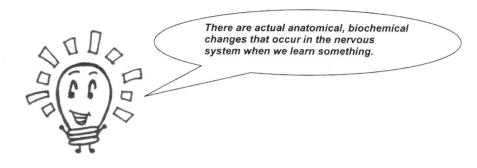

1. Imagine that a receiving neuron is at rest and not being stimulated. Imagine that some of the receptors on the receiving neuron (the baseball gloves described earlier), are somewhat hidden under the surface of the cell membrane. This is actually normal. Typically many receptors on the neuron cell membranes are hidden under the surface and are latent or waiting to be called into action. When the neuron is being stimulated, some of the hidden receptors come out to the surface of the neuron, resulting in more receptors ready to receive neurotransmitters (the baseballs).

2. The receptors on the surface of the cell membranes open up more to receive the neurotransmitter molecules more readily. Staying with our analogy, there are more baseball gloves out on the surface and they are more open and ready to catch and release baseballs.

3. The dendrites of the receiving, post-synaptic neuron flatten out and change their shape to allow more surface area to receive neurotransmitter molecules.

4. The receiving, post-synaptic neuron sends chemicals back to the pre-synaptic neuron to persuade this sending neuron to keep sending more of the stimulating chemicals. This is called *retrograde transmission*. These retrograde neurotransmitters are mainly gases, like *nitric oxide*. This is not the same as *nitrous oxide*, or *laughing gas*, which is used in the dentist's office. These retrograde neurotransmitters seem to encourage the sending neuron to send more of

its excitatory neurotransmitter, glutamate, to further facilitate learning. Glutamate is the main neurotransmitter that facilitates learning. It is the most abundant excitatory neurotransmitter in the nervous system. Too much glutamate excreted from over-stimulated and over-excited cells can result in the death of neurons. This is called **glutamatergic cytotoxicity**. This can occur in epilepsy, stroke, and other conditions that involve too much stimulation of the neurons for too long a time. This can also occur in the experience of long-term pain.

If a person is experiencing intense pain, he or she may also become more sensitive to other stimuli, such as loud sounds, sharp pinches, or even emotional experiences or thoughts. This phenomenon is called **sensitization**. It is an increase in response to mild stimuli as a result of previous exposure to more intense stimuli. This might be associated with glutamate cellular over-excitation. If something could be done to block glutamate excitatory over-activity, maybe pain could be lessened.

Olga described the pain of **Reflex Sympathetic Dystrophy (RSD)**, also referred to as **Complex Regional Pain Syndrome**. She had broken her right forearm and had several surgeries. She held the arm in a very guarded manner and was extremely sensitive to the lightest touch on the arm. She stated that the pain was burning, constant, nauseating, and severe. She described the fact that it felt much worse one time when she was passing a kidney stone. This might be an example of cooperativity and associativity, two stimuli paired together.

Anna had shoulder surgery and developed neuropathic pain around her shoulder. One day she spilled some hot coffee on her chest (not on her shoulder) and the neuropathic pain that she had around her shoulder was aggravated both subjectively and objectively by the hot coffee spill on her chest. We could see the skin around her shoulder redden very much like the hot burn area on her chest from the coffee. Again, this might be an example of cooperativity and associativity.

There are a lot of things that you can do to effect pain signals. If you always do what you always did, you'll always get what you always got. In order to change a painful experience, you may need to change the things you do, the thoughts you have, and your feelings as well. You may have to change the pathways and networks.

At the cellular level, learning and LTP is the process of making pathways in the nervous system work more readily and consistently. Changing the strength of synaptic communication is the basis of learning and LTP. Communication between neurons changes as a result of experience.

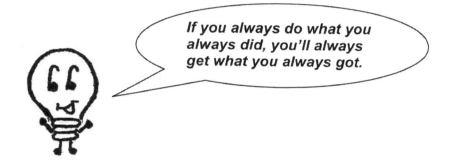

Neuroplasticity is the nervous system's ability to change or to learn by strengthening the connections already present, making new connections, making new organization of networks, and reorganizing itself anatomically and functionally. This also includes *neurogenesis*, which is the brain's ability to create new neurons. This only occurs in certain brain parts as far as is known.

Neuroplastic changes that originate from your own thoughts, feelings, decisions, behaviors and actions may be different than neuroplastic changes that occur or originate from something simply being done to you rather than done by you. *Locus of control* refers to a person's perception of control or responsibility for his or her own life and actions. If this sense of control originates from inside the person it is referred to as *internal locus of control*. A person may not feel a sense of control or may only be a passive participant in a situation. The person may be controlled by forces outside oneself. This is referred to as ***external locus of control.*** Sometimes people believe that the only way to bring about change is to have something done to them, like some formal medical intervention. Is it possible that something done internally could be even more powerful or give more long-term benefit as opposed to only temporary relief from passive therapies?

Frequently the person struggling with long-term pain is in a passive mode of functioning. This person receives massage, whirlpool, spinal manipulation, injections, and many other fairly passive approaches to pain relief and treatment. This person often experiences temporary relief at best. It is the gentle, active approaches like exercise, mental imagery, small steps to solve problems, and making efforts to learn new things that tend to give more long-term benefits. These active approaches may facilitate neuroplastic changes that are more lasting and helpful in the long run.

Forgetting, Long-Term Depression (LTD)

Wouldn't it be nice to be able to forget about a long-term painful experience? *Long-term depression, LTD*, does not refer to the emotional, cognitive, and behavioral condition of depression. It refers to biological occurrences at the cellular level: microscopic, biochemical, physiologic changes in the neurons and neuronal interactions. It refers to a prolonged decrease in response at a synapse. It occurs when axons have been inactive or only active at a low frequency. The person forgets; the nervous system forgets. When in pain, we forget how to be joyful and participate in gentle activities. We become less sensitive to pleasurable stimuli. Synapses with greater average activity become potentiated, or more easily excited. Those with less activity become depressed. This is "use it or lose it" at the cellular, synaptic level.

At the cellular level this is also called *down-regulation*. This is essentially the opposite of up-regulation or long-term potentiation. This is actually what happens with tolerance to medications over time. The person starts to need more and more of the medication to do the same job. Since some neuronal pathways are constantly or repetitively bombarded by opioid chemicals introduced into the nervous system from the outside, the internal endorphin chemical system is quieted, not used, and down-regulated.

The receptors in the post-synaptic neuron of the internal endorphin/opioid system withdraw somewhat inside the cell membrane. The ones remaining on the surface tend to close up somewhat, becoming less ready and able to receive or catch the neurotransmitter or opioid molecules. The dendrites change their shape again and are less capable of receiving the neurotransmitters. The retrograde transmission is lessened. All of this facilitates less learning, and in fact, more forgetting. These are neuroplastic changes that sometimes are not so helpful.

People dealing with long-term pain have often expressed how the medical system, the worker's compensation system, and the personal injury system can be extremely stressful. Pain itself is stressful as well. Perpetual stress in these systems may cause abnormal neuroplastic changes in the nervous system. In the worker's compensation system, many times the only way the patient can get help is to complain or get worse with respect to their symptoms. Of course, one does not usually get worse on purpose, but getting worse does often get positive reinforcement in terms of further medical care and attention. Getting worse can also lessen the forced involvement in a situation which hurts more, such as a particular work situation. Coming to settlement in the medical/legal system might allow for other more beneficial and calming neuroplastic changes to occur in the long run.

A thirty-eight year old man, Alfonso, had low back pain and leg pain ever since a work injury two years before. He also underwent L5-S1 laminectomy, discectomy without much benefit. He understood that ongoing pain was associated with scar tissue on the nerve. He stated, "Since I have had so much pain for so long, my body seems to be less sensitive to pain. I could put a nail through my hand. It doesn't bother me like it did. This is the way things are. It doesn't have to run my life." He continued to work full time, care for his family, and did fairly well with minimal medication use.

How is it that some people with long-term pain experience more sensitivity to other stimuli, and some experience less sensitivity to stimuli, painful or otherwise? What neuroplastic changes occur in a person's brain/body associated with settling things in his own mind? What mental and physical activities can be practiced in order to do and be as healthy and well as one can be?

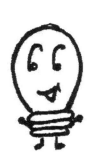

It might be easier to let go of something if one is grabbing a hold of something else.

Habituation is similar to long-term depression. Habituation is a decrease in response to a stimulus that is presented repeatedly. The bears in Yellowstone Park habituate to people and cars. They don't respond much to their presence. Long-term depression is a decrease in synaptic activity and it is associated with disuse. It can also be associated with overuse. When using opioids for pain relief, certain neurologic pathways are stimulated over and over until they require more and more stimulus to get the same response. The person becomes tolerant, almost immune, to the medication. The over medicated pathways become habituated to the medication. They become insensitive to the medication. The same biological processes occur as described above. The receptors in the post-synaptic neuron withdraw somewhat inside the cell membrane. Those remaining on the surface tend to close up somewhat, becoming less ready and able to receive or catch the neurotransmitter or opioid molecules. The dendrites change their shape and are less capable of receiving the neurotransmitters. The retrograde transmission is lessened. These neuroplastic changes are not so helpful.

One might hope for habituation when dealing with long-term pain. One might hope that we would just get used to the pain and not notice it so much. But sometimes simply ignoring it might lead to other problems. A patient described, "I tried to teach myself to not be startled by a noise or stimulus. I tried to suppress my emotions." He wondered if this resulted in hypersensitivity. He said, "I might not startle so much, but I would *jump to weird conclusions.*" The sound of a squirrel in the attic would make him think of many animals setting up home and he would catastrophize, or think the worst, think that the house would crumble. Rather than simply ignoring something, one might retrain the nervous system to be involved and active in something else. It might be easier to let go of something if one is grabbing a hold of something else.

Sometimes the person might then tend to over-think and may not feel normal emotions, or they may not let themselves feel normal emotions. The person in pain might not allow the feeling of depression because of not wanting to appear depressed. The person might not allow happiness because they think that when someone is in pain they shouldn't feel happy.

Raymond, sixty years old, described being hurt on the job ten years earlier. He subsequently underwent two neck surgeries and two low back surgeries. He had not worked in many years. He described the support that he experienced from his family and friends, his church, and his faith. He also stated that, "I sometimes call it a silent pain. My body is reacting unconsciously. My body knows the pain is there, even though my mind and heart are managing it well, or so I think. I get ulcers, muscle tightness, and my shaking picks up. I meditate so I don't sense it, but my body is still dealing with it. I tend to deal with it little bits at a time, to take the edge off." At times his legs gave out and he felt "electric shocks" through his "whole body." What could he do differently to facilitate more consistent calm, happiness, and peace? Taking medications might lessen the pain, but calming emotions might provide a more lasting change.

A person may need to make new paths in the nervous system by practicing something other than suppression of emotions. When the person feels angry, he may need to say to himself that this feeling is a good and normal thing. It is natural and understandable.

He may need to learn new strategies and techniques to manage this anger and associated pain . Who knows what will work? It has been said that doing the same thing over and over and expecting a different outcome is a definition of insanity.

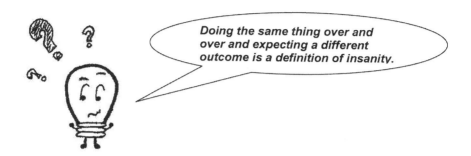

Another patient said, "Coping is minimizing some things sometimes, and maximizing some things other times. I can adjust my thinking and behaviors. I am doing the work of a track official at auto races. Sometimes it is too hard to focus. I tend to fidget because of the leg pain. I have a failed back surgery and nerve damage into my leg. I can't do the work as well as I would like and I am concerned about what others think. Because of the pain sometimes it seems ten times harder just to try to function normally."

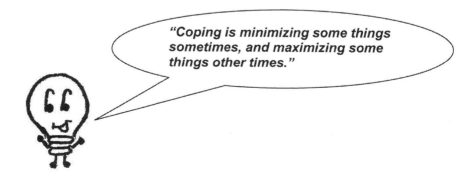

Another patient described his behavior and effects on other people. He felt he was driving all his friends and relatives away. He said, "It might be like walking down the street with a broken toe. Everybody looks at you funny, like why is he walking that way? Or they all feel sorry for you. Pain behaviors might drive others away. Walking down the street just after finding a $100 bill would be different and might attract people. You would be all excited, and everybody would want to know why."

Joyce, a forty-five year old woman with fibromyalgia-like syndrome, an L3-4 focal paracentral disc herniation, degenerative disc problems in her neck, and headaches, said, "I've been told I have 'vasovagal syncope' with my pain. This seems to happen when I lay down. All of my organs seem to shut down, and it feels like all the blood goes to my brain. Suddenly I get nausea, and sometimes vomiting and diarrhea. My eyes roll back; I lose consciousness; I have low blood pressure and at other times my blood pressure is high. I constantly feel like I just finished the flu; I'm drained and fatigued." What can she change? How can she think, feel, and behave differently?

A very psychologically minded patient asked, "Can pain itself become an anti-anxiety medication? Can pain be an unconscious way of avoiding things? It is clear that a variety of experiences and conditions can alter the experience or phenomenon of pain. Opioids, marijuana, many other medications, exercise, meditation, might all make pain worse or better. Anxiety, fear, and anger might make pain worse, but can they also be pain reducers?"

Another gentleman, a seventy-five year old ex-fighter pilot and ship captain, described his fear by stating, "I have more fear with pain than when in a burning building. I'm tough. I'm a pilot. I could nose dive an airplane to a hundred feet from the ground and then pull up. I am more afraid of the pain than of that. I was captain of ships in fifty to sixty foot waves. I'm more afraid of pain than of that. I've kayaked in class six waters. I'm more afraid of pain than of that. I'm more afraid of coming off thirty-five mg of Oxycodone per day than I was of any of those experiences." What can he do and how can we help him to change his thoughts, feelings, and behaviors and be successful in his situation?

Pain is very complicated, multifaceted, and experienced uniquely by each individual person. There are many brain parts, networks, and chemicals involved in the painful experience. There are certain parts and networks that are extremely significant. These include the amygdala, hippocampus, hypothalamus, pituitary gland, adrenal glands, anterior cingulate cortex, frontal lobe, and many other structures that interact with each other and are constantly changing. These parts, networks, and interactions can be changed for the better. They can be modified to make a difference in the painful experience.

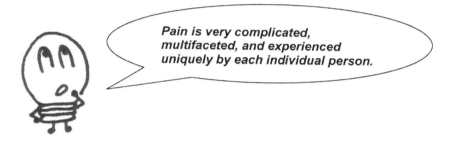

Pain is very complicated, multifaceted, and experienced uniquely by each individual person.

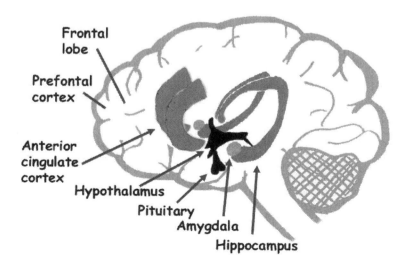

Amygdala

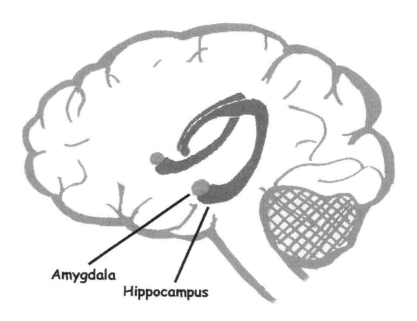

Amygdala means "almond." It is shaped like an almond and is located on both sides of the brain, deep in the base and temporal areas. It is part of the limbic system where we experience powerful feelings or emotions. Limbic means "border". It is the border between higher cortical areas (surface or cortex, or neocortex as described in the triune brain) and deeper areas of the brain (the reptilian brain comprised of the brain stem and the cerebellum).

The amygdala is considered to be the seat of emotional memories, particularly fear and anxiety or other uncomfortable feelings. It is associated with the deep feelings one might experience when in danger. It is also involved in experiencing many other emotions, including joy, peace, love, excitement, and other positive emotions. Many brain parts and networks are involved in emotions. There are no exclusively specific, localized places for anger or depression or happiness. There are, rather, networks of brain parts involved in these experiences. Emotions are extremely complex. Longing to see a grown daughter who has moved far away is different than nostalgia when thinking about your high school athletic accomplishments.

The amygdala is not only involved in emotions, but also in decision making. In fact, the amygdala and its emotional sensitivity, memory, and expression is more involved in decision making than some other parts of the brain that specialize in logic and reason. The amygdala is active when we have a hunch or a gut-feeling or "women's intuition" about something.

It is very hard to make decisions without emotional input. For example, we need and use the amygdala to decide which valentine's card to buy. We look through all the cards in the store. From a practical, logical standpoint, they are all very similar with black words and red hearts. But then one tickles your fancy, makes you chuckle or feel good, and you think your loved one might also like it. You are familiar with what your loved one might like; you are familiar with what tickles the amygdala of your loved one. Your amygdalae resonate together, figuratively speaking. The emotional content of the valentine's card experience is at least in part due to the activity in the amygdala.

When we say some brain structure is active at a certain time, we mean that during testing, such as *fMRI (functional magnet resonance imaging)* or *PET scan (Positron Emission Tomography)*, this area of the brain lights up during a particular activity. For example, the amygdala lights up during deep prayer. The person in the fMRI machine is asked to pray deeply. The machine measures the activity of oxygen utilization in the brain parts at that time. The amygdala utilizes oxygen more than other brain parts during deep prayer.

TV violence activates the amygdala. When a person is watching TV violence, the amygdala activates, uses more oxygen, and lights up on the fMRI.

Emotions can be very intense and even explosive. They can be experienced overtly, clearly, and obviously. However, they can also sometimes be experienced on a subconscious or unconscious level. Emotions can be very subtle, slow in developing, short-term or long-term. You may experience emotions but not really be aware of them. You may feel something but not really be clear about what you are feeling. You may not be aware of why you are feeling the way you do or what is causing the emotions or feelings.

The amygdala reacts to faces depicting emotions such as fear, deceit, anxiety, anger, and tension even on a subconscious, intuitive level. A person can watch a TV screen as various facial expressions are flashed on the screen so fast that the person doesn't even know that they are faces, or at least does not recognize any particular emotions in the faces. But when the faces express fear or terror, the amygdala lights up. Again, the person viewing the screen may not even be consciously aware of the fact that facial expressions are being presented. Yet the amygdala, on a subconscious level, is aware, sensitive, and responsive. It lights up with increased metabolic activity.

The amygdala helps in recognition of facial expression and tones of voice. A child or a person who doesn't know the language can still recognize and feel the emotion in the tone of a person's voice. If the voice or facial expression is subtle enough, the person may not be aware, on a conscious level, of the emotional content of the voice, faces, or experiences. But the person may still register the emotional information on a subconscious level.

An article on the brain in the March 2005 issue of National Geographic magazine commented, "Highly emotional memories etched in the amygdala may not be accessible to the conscious mind, but still influence how we act and feel beyond our awareness." Our subconscious feelings influence our conscious decisions all the time.

The amygdala can be hypersensitive and hyperreactive. This might be due to the long-term, even life-long, inputs of stressful, anxiety producing experiences. It might be due to more acute or recent difficult struggles in life. Repetitive and long-term anxiety producing experiences or intense, acute anxiety producing experiences may stimulate the amygdala in such a way that it becomes extremely sensitive and ready to respond at the slightest stimulus. Its responses send messages of alarm throughout the brain and body.

Rats that are repeatedly exposed to light followed by a shock soon show a startle reflex when simply exposed to the light. This is called a priming effect. The amygdala becomes very sensitive to a stimulus that is paired with the shock. This connection will continue unless something is done to change the situation.

An area of the brain that tends to calm down the amygdala is the *pre-frontal cortex (PFC)*. The PFC, the front part of the brain, governs logical, reasonable, rational thinking, and is used for foresight and planning about the future. This area of the brain can help look ahead and think about what is important in life at this specific time as well as in the future. It can help plan small steps to solve problems. It helps interpret and analyze information and make decisions about responses and meanings to events and experiences. It is in charge of executive functions. When it comes to decision making, it is part of your conscience; it helps you know right from wrong and helps you to do the right thing.

There are projections or nerve pathways from the pre-frontal cortex to the amygdala. This allows logical, practical thinking processes to calm down emotional decision making. Interestingly, in general, there are more projections or nerve pathways from the amygdala to the prefrontal cortex. Thus, sometimes emotions may have a bigger role to play in one's decision-making processes.

Adults tend to use the PFC to identify and interpret facial expressions. Adolescents tend to use the amygdala. If a friend at school makes a face at the adolescent, the adolescent may experience significant emotion and tend to interpret and respond in a very emotional manner. If a person is driving and is cut off or honked at by another driver, the adult may simply drive on and not get too emotional or bent out of shape. The adolescent, using his or her amygdala mostly, or the adult who is not using his or her PFC very well, may go into road rage.

The amygdala is rich in receptors for testosterone. Young males with higher levels of testosterone may experience more emotion in their daily activities, as the amygdala may be more stimulated by higher levels of testosterone. Essentially, this is a priming effect as well, making the amygdala more sensitive to stimuli and more ready to respond. Testosterone does not cause emotional lability or instability. Testosterone does not cause a person to respond emotionally or violently. It does, however, cause the amygdala to become somewhat more sensitive and ready to respond emotionally.

Much of the information about brain parts and networks is learned because of the work done on animals. We extrapolate to people and observe the same or similar behaviors. A mouse may learn to avoid a part of the environment where it has been given a shock in the past. It may avoid related or similar parts of the environment. The animal or person may be more anxious when exposed to particular environmental stimuli that somehow relate to the environment where it was shocked. This phenomenon is called *learned-shock-avoidance*. This accounts for many forms of anxiety.

Benzodiazepines are medications that typically lessen anxiety. They are also called tranquilizers or anxiolytics. As with all medications, benzodiazepines go almost everywhere in the brain/body, but much of their beneficial activity is in the amygdala and *hypothalamus*. Benzodiazepines decrease learned-shock-avoidance. They lessen avoidance behavior. An animal or a person, when given these chemicals, will be less cautious in approaching the various environmental stimuli.

The same is true of humans using benzodiazepines or any chemicals, such as alcohol, that calm the amygdala. If a person is afraid of dogs because he or she was bitten once, benzodiazepines might lessen the anxiety associated with seeing dogs, hearing dogs, or being near dogs. Benzodiazepines are used to decrease many anxiety disorders including phobias, panic attacks, generalized anxiety disorder, post-traumatic stress disorder, and others.

Benzodiazepines go to the amygdala and hypothalamus to increase social interactions with unfamiliar partners. Sometimes the benzodiazepines can be used to lessen social phobia, fear or anxiety, and the tendency to avoid specific social or performance situations. Because the emotional alarm system of anxiety, fear, and caution might not work as well as it should when benzodiazepines are used, the person or animal may be less inhibited or more willing to be involved in unfamiliar social interactions.

Benzodiazepines act in the amygdala and hypothalamus to increase muscle relaxation or decrease muscle tightness. For example, Valium, or the generic name diazepam, is not only an anxiolytic or tranquilizer but also a muscle relaxer.

Benzodiazepines are sometimes used to prevent seizures or abnormal electrical activity in the brain. Sometimes they may have a peripheral effect on abnormal nerve impulses. Both the central and peripheral effects of these agents can alter the unpleasantness of a painful experience.

Activity in the amygdala is typically high during sleep. Think of the emotional content of dreams. Sometimes people have nightmares, but even when dreams are pleasant they are often packed with emotion. You might try to remember details about a dream: the scenes, characters, and facts. Sometimes this is difficult. However, the emotional content is often more easily remembered. It can also be enlightening to think about the emotional content of your dreams.

Bipolar patients, in general, have a larger than normal amygdala. The depression phases and the manic phases are intensely emotional. The person experiencing these may have difficulty thinking clearly and may use emotion more than they would like in their daily activities, decision-making, and behaviors.

We have seen what happens when the amygdala is hyperactive or over stimulated. What happens if the amygdala is damaged or destroyed in such a way that it becomes less sensitive and reactive to stimuli?

One condition associated with significant damage to the amygdala is known as **Kluver-Bucy syndrome**. It results in less fear of people, experiences, or situations than one ought to have in order to maintain safety. Some caution in new relationships can be warranted as not all people are trustworthy. Damage to the amygdala may result in less caution and care. This can be just like the effects of tranquilizers, alcohol, and benzodiazepines which dull or inhibit the amygdala and result in less caution and care.

Another condition is ***Urbach-Weithe disease***, a rare genetic disorder in which the amygdala is calcified. There is minimal emotional awareness or response to normal life experiences. This might be likened to the TV character in Star Trek named Data. He was a computer that looked like a man but had no feelings or emotions.

The amygdala, or its pathways and network connections, can also be damaged by stroke, trauma, tumor, chemical damage, or infection. This can result in the same type of non-emotional experience and expression. The person may lack empathy and sympathy in various situations after significant damage to the amygdala or its networks.

One might wonder about the person with antisocial personality disorder, who may lack empathy and remorse after destructive behavior. The Diagnostic and Statistical Manual, Fourth Edition, Text Revision (DSM-IV-TR) of the American Psychiatric Association lists the classic descriptive characteristics of this disorder. These include the general characteristics of "intense emotional experience and expression, poor impulse control, and poor frustration tolerance."

Does this person experience emotions intensely in some situations and minimally or not at all in others? Is this learned? Has the amygdala been trained to be sensitive in some situations and insensitive and unresponsive in others? Is this similar to all of us in some ways? Are we sensitive to some situations and issues and insensitive to others? Can we learn and be trained to think and feel differently?

If you find yourself anxious, tense, crying, irritable, on edge, short tempered, or sad for no reason, it may be that your amygdala, among other things, is primed like a pump or motor and is ready to function fully. This can be good in terms of safety, but it can be too sensitive or too responsive.

The ***Moro response*** of a newborn infant may also be an example. When the infant is exposed to a loud sound or shaking of the crib, the baby's arms, legs, neck, and head extend and suddenly become very stiff. This is an automatic protective response. The sudden sound or stimulation travels rapidly through the brain and down to the pons, the middle of the brainstem. Then the message travels immediately out to the peripheral nerves of the body, particularly to the muscles around the neck and the shoulders. The muscles in the neck and body become instantly tight and tense to protect the infant.

In adulthood this similar neurological network might also account for some of the ongoing and significant neck, shoulder, and head muscle tightness that occurs when people are under extra stress and strain in their lives. Normally in adulthood our higher cortical functions can calm and put a damper on this automatic response to stressful stimuli. The brand-new infant's higher cortical functions are not fully developed and thus are not able to put a damper on the reflexes. In adulthood, when the amygdala is too hypersensitive and too hyperreactive, the higher cortical functions of the brain may not be up to the task of emotional inhibition.

My wife and I attended the movie *Omen* many years ago. It was a very frightening movie at the time. When we came out of the movie theater and held hands as we walked down the dark street, I leaned over to my wife and said, "Boo." She jumped, terrified, and I actually jumped as well. I think I scared myself. We were both so tense, hyper-vigilant, frightened, and on the edge from the movie that our normal, natural startle response was primed, heightened, and exaggerated.

This readiness and response are biochemical phenomena in the brain and body. Our bodies manufacture and utilize a chemical called *cholecystokinin (CCK)*. This chemical is a stimulating drug for the amygdala. If one injects stimulating drugs into the amygdala, the startle response is exaggerated and increased.

The hyperactive startle response of *Post-Traumatic-Stress-Disorder (PTSD)* is an example of the primed amygdala. The person is hyper-vigilant and on edge. It doesn't take much stimulus for the amygdala to be activated and to send messages throughout the brain/body. It is interesting to know that in PTSD there can be actual waxing and waning between emotional hypersensitivity (too emotional) and psychic numbing (minimal emotions). It may be that the amygdala needs a periodic break in order to function more normally.

Hippocampus

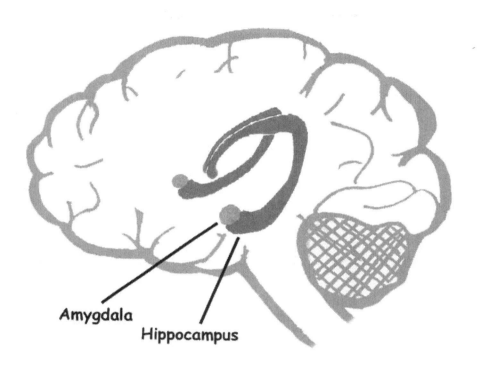

Amygdala

Hippocampus

Janet, a patient with a worker's compensation injury and long-term pain, is living in the residential rehabilitation facility to help learn better ways to deal with chronic pain. This is a three week in-patient comprehensive, multi-disciplinary pain management program designed not so much for lessening pain, but rather for helping people increase function and life. It helps people with a pain problem that cannot be fixed to learn different ways of coping and to live better with what they have by focusing not just on the pain but also on their strengths.

Janet comes out of her room one morning at about 9:10 and says, in an angry, frantic and emotional voice, "I've locked myself out of my room two times already this morning, and left my watch down in the pool area. I'm in my soaking wet bathing suit and it is very upsetting." She is not thinking clearly and is acting or behaving with extreme emotion. One might think in biological terms and wonder what parts and networks of her brain, nervous system, and body are involved in this process. One might wonder what chemicals are involved or "out of balance."

One brain part to consider is the hippocampus. It is a part of the limbic system as is the amygdala. The hippocampus is a part of the brain located inside the temporal lobes on both sides of the brain. Humans and other animals have two hippocampi, one in each side of the brain. The name derives from its curved shape, which resembles a seahorse. In Greek "hippo" means "horse" and "campus" means "sea monster."

Psychologists and neuroscientists in general agree that the hippocampus is central in the formation, recording, and encoding of new memories. This is particularly true about experienced episodes and events. These are called episodic or autobiographical memories.

There are two main types of memories:

1. **Declarative/explicit/autobiographical/conscious**

    a.   **Semantic memory**
    b.   **Episodic memory**

2. **Procedural/implicit/emotional/unconscious**

Declarative or explicit memory is more conscious memory. Declarative means memories that can be explicitly verbalized or declared out loud. These would include, for example, memory of facts, the details of episodes, or autobiographical or personal experiences.

This type of memory has two subcategories. The first is semantic memory. This is not memory about a specific event, but rather the meaning of things. For example, you are asked the question, "Are dogs animals or people?" You may not remember a specific event or learning episode or the specific time that you learned this fact, but you do know the meaning and the answer to this question.

The second declarative or explicit memory is called episodic memory. This is specific memory about events, times, and places. I remember what I had for breakfast this morning. I remember what we did for Christmas last year. I remember what I was doing when 9/11 occurred.

The second main type of memory is called procedural or implicit memory. This is more unconscious. It involves skills such as tying your shoes, riding a bike, using silverware, reading, writing, playing the piano, singing, and many other similar things. It also involves emotional memories: feeling particular emotions when exposed to a particular stimulus. This exposure may be through any of our senses, thoughts, emotions, and even painful stimuli.

Janet was having problems with her hippocampus. It was not functioning normally. She was not thinking clearly. She wondered if she was getting *Alzheimer's disease.*

In Alzheimer's disease the hippocampus is one of the first regions of the brain to suffer damage. The general cortex, and particularly the frontal lobe, deteriorates gradually as well. Memory problems and disorientation appear first. Damage to the hippocampus can occur for many reasons. Degeneration is one of those reasons which can occur with gradual dying, shrinking, and atrophy of the cells. Damage can also result from many other pathologic conditions such as a lack of oxygen, inflammation, infection, stroke, or tumor. Significant and severe stress can also be one of these causes. Pain and its effects are stressful and can cause hippocampal damage.

Many memories often last a lifetime. It is felt that long-term memory is based on consolidation of memory. The broad definition of *memory consolidation* is the process by which recent memories are crystallized into long-term memory. Consolidation implies sending information from the hippocampus to various other parts of the brain, particularly to various parts of the cortex or surface of the brain, for long-term storage and retrieval as needed.

Some evidence supports the idea that the hippocampus ceases to play a crucial role in the retention of some memories after a period of consolidation. This process of consolidation, at the molecular/cellular level, involves the strengthening of synapses between neurons of the hippocampus and other brain parts and networks. Eventually the hippocampus may not be as involved in long-term, well consolidated memories. But it is extremely important in the formation of new memories.

All memory, at the molecular level, requires protein synthesis and utilization of the proteins in the nervous system. Remember that proteins are important for all functions of the brain/body. The changes at the molecular level are called *molecular consolidation*. This is what happens in the nervous system. There are also similar changes throughout the rest of the body. There is a brain/ body connection when we remember things. There is never a brain/body separation. You probably have heard the term *muscle memory*. The muscle movements of the athlete or musician have become automatic. This is true for all of us in our normal activities of daily living. It is not really just in the muscles. It is in the brain/ body connection. Whenever we think or feel something, the body is also involved in the experience. Most of this involvement is unconscious. We are not necessarily aware of what is happening in the body. Also, whenever we experience something in the body, the brain and the rest of the nervous system is involved. Again, this is mostly on an unconscious level. This is true of pain as well. We experience it in the body but the whole brain/body connection is occurring without our conscious awareness.

What we experience unconsciously can become conscious. This can occur when we focus and pay attention to certain aspects of a situation, or if the experience is intense enough, such as with pain. This also might occur when a person experiences something and then thinks "this makes me think of something else." If you walk through the halls of your elementary school, not having set foot in the building for forty years, the sights and smells may cause you to experience all kinds of memories and thoughts and feelings. Those memories were stored in various places in your brain/body. If you pay attention to all of this, you might become more aware and more conscious of what was once unconscious, deeply stored, learned long ago, and really never forgotten.

Intense emotional content in a situation also adds to the phenomenon of consolidation and long-term consolidation. We know about being able to remember certain events because there was such intense emotion at the time, like knowing where you were when John F. Kennedy was shot or when the space shuttle Challenger blew up.

Consolidation occurs with repeated exposure to stimulus-response pairs. Consolidation increases in strength over time with repetition. Practice makes perfect. Maximum consolidation is achieved by means of *spaced repetition*. An example might be practicing a particularly difficult measure of music on the piano ten minutes a day for six days in a row, rather than sixty minutes all in one day. The brain/body memorization of this measure of music will be more successful with the spaced repetition.

Also, it typically is very difficult to start playing a memorized piece of piano music somewhere in the middle of the piece. We all know that typically the pianist has to start at the beginning of the piece or the beginning of a particular section. A stimulus, the beginning of the part, prompts a response in the nervous system and the body. The response of playing the next series of notes becomes another stimulus, which prompts another response, which becomes another stimulus, and so on. The pianist plays through the piece, all the parts flowing one after the other, in a very orderly fashion.

The person experiencing pain is similar to the pianist. The person learns various stimulus/response/stimulus/response thoughts, feelings, and behaviors mostly on an unconscious level. These patterns play over and over until they are hard to change. They are hardwired, so to speak. They are brain/body unconscious experiences that need to be brought to consciousness, at least partly, in order to work on changing the patterns.

Persons struggling with long-term pain basically do the same things in response to the flare-ups of pain every day. Patients have described staying horizontal and on medications until they feel a little better. Then they look around their home and see all the things that need to be done, since they haven't done anything while laying around and resting. Then they get up to do some of those things, since they feel better from lying around. But they tend to do too much, since they feel good enough and aren't sure when they will feel good enough again. In doing too much, they become flared-up with more pain. They then take another pill and go to bed to rest until they feel better. Once they feel better, they again see all the things that need to be done. They get up and do too much until they are flared-up again, and take a pill and go back to bed. This pattern continues, unchanged. This is learned behavior that becomes unrecognized for what it is until it is pointed out to the person. Then there are choices to be made, such as to continue to be an expert at the vicious cycle or practice significant changes.

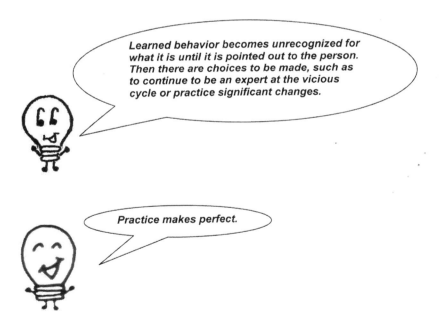

Learned behavior becomes unrecognized for what it is until it is pointed out to the person. Then there are choices to be made, such as to continue to be an expert at the vicious cycle or practice significant changes.

Practice makes perfect.

This process of consolidation begins during wakefulness and may be enhanced during sleep. Originally, it was thought that this happens during dreaming, or the **REM (rapid eye movements** *stages of sleep*). However, other research indicates that the NREM phases (or non-REM sleep) are associated with the process of consolidation as well. The person in pain often does not sleep well. Consolidation and memory difficulties are often problematic for the person with long-term pain.

"If you always do what you always did, you will always get what you always got." My family and I went to a resort for one week every summer for almost twenty years. There was free golf all week at the nine hole par three course adjoining the resort. I usually golfed five to six rounds every day. Each summer, when we returned home from the vacation, there was a par three golf tournament sponsored through our church. I had always imagined winning, or at least doing very well at the tournament, since I practiced twenty-five to thirty rounds during the week before. However, I always did lousy. I think this is because during the week of practice, I hit mostly lousy shots. I basically practiced lousy shots. I became an expert at lousy shots. I played in the tournament like I practiced during the vacation week, mainly just for fun.

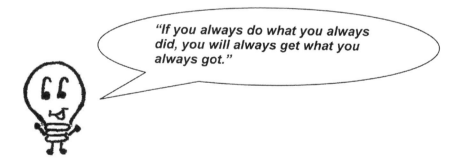

"If you always do what you always did, you will always get what you always got."

The person needs to retrain the brain and body to find a middle ground between doing too much and doing too little. This is often very difficult, but not impossible. The middle ground might be a moving target, in that some days are better or worse than others. The pattern and neurobiological pathways of stimulus-response need to be changed. This can happen with practice.

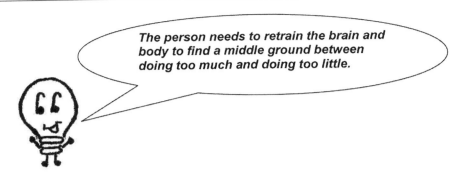

Not only are there different types of memory, there are also different types of forgetting.

1. *Anterograde amnesia*: Trouble forming new memories (for example, after an injury.)
2. *Retrograde amnesia*: Trouble accessing memories already present (for example, prior to an injury.)

Damage to the hippocampus usually results in profound difficulties in forming new memories. This is called ***anterograde amnesia***. In this form of memory loss, new events are not transferred to long-term memory. After the onset of the disorder, the person will not be able to recall events which occurred only moments earlier. Once attention has shifted to something else the person will not be able to remember what was going on previously.

Damage to the hippocampus can also affect access to memories prior to the damage. This is called ***retrograde amnesia***. Retrograde amnesia can extend back years prior to the brain damage. However, older memories may remain. The sparing of older memories leads further to the idea that consolidation over time involves the transfer of memories out of the hippocampus to other parts of the brain/body.

Damage to the hippocampus does not affect some aspects of memory. This might include the ability to learn new skills such as playing a musical instrument. This suggests that such abilities depend on the other type of memory, the procedural memory, as described above. This type of memory involves different brain/ body regions and networks.

Some research indicates that even if the hippocampi are damaged severely, semantic memory may still be intact. Semantic memory may be partially located in structures around the hippocampus called ***parahippocampal*** nuclei. Semantic memories are distributed in multiple cortical brain structures and networks. For example, the memory of the sound of a dog barking might be located in the auditory cortex. The memory of the site of the dog might be located in the visual cortex.

Some evidence implicates the hippocampus in storing and processing spatial memory and navigational information. Studies with rats have shown that neurons in the hippocampus have spatial firing fields. These cells are called ***place cells***. Place cells have now been seen in humans. They are actively firing when the person is finding his or her way around in a virtual reality situation. These findings resulted from research with individuals that had electrodes implanted in their brains as a diagnostic part of surgical treatment for serious epilepsy.

The hippocampus probably does not act as a cognitive map or a neural representation of the layout of the environment. It may be crucial for more fundamental processes within navigation. Studies with animals have shown that an intact hippocampus is required for simple spatial memory tasks such as finding the way back to a hidden goal.

Without a fully functioning hippocampus, humans may not successfully remember where they have been and how to get where they are going. Researchers believe that the hippocampus plays a particularly important role in finding short cuts between familiar places. Some people exhibit more skill at this sort of navigation than do others, and brain imaging shows that these individuals have more active hippocampi when navigating.

London taxi drivers must learn a large number of places and know the most direct routes between them. They have to pass a strict test, called "the knowledge", before being licensed to drive the cabs. A study at University College London showed that part of the hippocampus is larger in taxi drivers than in the general public and that more experienced drivers have bigger hippocampi.

It should be noted that alcohol disrupts learning and long term potentiation significantly, particularly in the hippocampus. In general, the hippocampi are smaller in heavy alcohol users. More specifically, if you drink too much on a particular evening, you may not remember much of the events of that night.

Remember Janet, the patient who kept losing her keys? Her hippocampus was not working well and she was extremely emotional about her situation. Her hippocampus was under stress and had been in this predicament for a long time. She was not able to think clearly. She also had trouble controlling emotional responses. Her amygdala was hypersensitive and hyperreactive to extremes of emotional experience and expression. This is sometimes called *emotion dysregulation*. She tended to approach everything from a very emotional standpoint. She had a long history of anger at the particular perceived injustices in her worker's compensation situation. She had a long history of anger, anxiety, and depression associated with her perception that her medical care had been poor. The history actually went back even further. She stated that she was abused in childhood and experienced what she felt was poor treatment associated with childhood polio. She also experienced a sense of injustice in her work place for many years, even before her injury. She stated, "I gave the place 150 percent. They never really appreciated me. It took three people to replace me when I couldn't work there anymore."

One hour after her complaints about misplacing her keys she came in screaming that she had now lost her keys for the third time that morning. She has practiced, and has become an expert at, being emotional and extreme in her own feelings and responses to stress and distress in her life.

An emotionally upset patient calls about not being able to obtain his opioids as he believes he should. He calls three times before he leaves his phone number for us to return his call. We return his call and in a tense, heavy, anxious, breathy voice he states he is having withdrawal symptoms and increased pain since using up his medications early and running out. He is struggling emotionally. He states that he feels his blood pressure is high. His amygdala is working overtime in terms of his emotional experience. His hippocampus is having trouble thinking clearly. Our response is to give some medication for withdrawal symptoms which calms the amygdala slightly and can lower blood pressure, and eventually we all hope that his hippocampus will come around to normal again. Wouldn't it be best if he could make some changes in his own perceptions, responses, and behaviors to help facilitate this process?

At the introductions for involvement in the pain management program one of the patients stated, "I can't think this morning." He was trying to answer simple questions to give some basic introductory information about himself. He was simply trying to state his name, where he was from, his favorite plant, and the last thing that he read. He was having trouble with simple basic information. His hippocampus was in trouble.

The hippocampus and amygdala can be in conflict. The logical reasoning functions and the emotional functions can be contradictory. The emotional side of things can be so heightened that it is difficult to think clearly.

As stated earlier, the amygdala is a key brain region in processing emotions. It is essential in interpreting and integrating emotions, particularly emotions related to anxiety and fear. The amygdala is one main area where fear learned from past experience is stored. The amygdala plays a central role in processing emotional colors or flavors (so to speak) attached to all external and internal experiences, thoughts, feelings, behaviors, and information. It is central to all afferent (incoming) and efferent (outgoing) connections related to emotional functioning. This means that it is central to, and applies emotional color or flavor to, all the messages that enter into the brain and all the messages that exit from the brain.

The amygdala receives input from various systems throughout the brain and the body. It processes the emotional value or context related to the inputs. These inputs can be simple or very complex, and come from many different brain/body areas and systems including complex multi-sensory, cognitive, behavioral, autonomic, and neuroendocrine systems.

Let's return to our earlier example about picking out a valentine's card. You have found one that you really like, one that tickles your fancy, or probably tickles your amygdala. You turn the card over and see that it is $45.12. Your hippocampus and frontal lobe say, "No, we are not getting this one; it is too expensive." But your amygdala says, "Yes, but this one is so good and so funny; I want this one." So your reason and emotion are in some conflict.

Typically, until you are twenty-five years old or so, your amygdala and its emotion laden projections are often more powerful than your frontal lobe and hippocampus in decision making. By early adulthood your frontal lobe becomes more developed and more in control in decision making. For many people, when "push comes to shove," we will make decisions based on emotions. If we cannot decide based on the facts, if we cannot decide based on the lists of pros and cons, priorities, or the consequences of our actions, we will decide based on emotions.

There are many other brain/body parts and networks involved in the experience of pain. A person with chronic pain may have an overactive amygdala and a hippocampus that can't calm the anxious person down. The amygdala and hippocampus try to influence other brain parts and each other. One brain part that is extremely important is the hypothalamus.

Hypothalamus

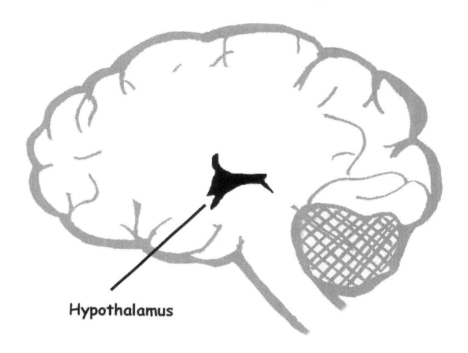

Hypothalamus

The hypothalamus is a small part of the brain made of many nuclei or smaller parts. It controls many functions including the brain/body responses to *acute stress*, fight or flight. This involves immediate electrical neural transmissions. The hypothalamus also manufactures and secretes many hormones into the blood stream for more long-term use. This is part of the problems and solutions associated with *long-term stress*.

The amygdala and the hippocampus, along with all the other structures of the limbic system, constantly try to influence the hypothalamus and its functions. For example, the amygdala, with its emotional intensity and sometimes dysregulation, tries to convince the hypothalamus to continue emotional commotion and upheaval. The hippocampus and the frontal lobes, at the same time, try to facilitate more calm and reason in the situation by sending inhibitory, calming messages to the amygdala and logic, reason, and thought into the hypothalamus. In turn, the hypothalamus sends messages to the pituitary gland.

Pituitary

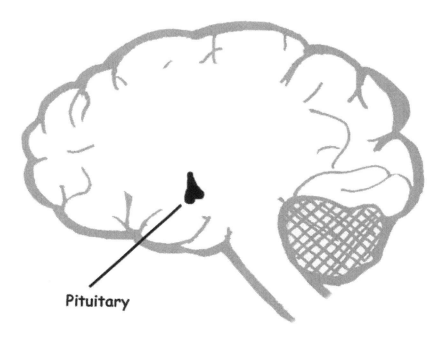

Pituitary

The pituitary gland is about the size of a pea, yet it has been called "the master gland" because of its influence on all the hormonal systems of the brain/body. In reality, there is no master gland as such. The pituitary is very important but it is only part of a larger system of hormonal control which includes all the structures of the brain/body. The pituitary gland influences many organs of the body. We will focus on the adrenal glands.

Adrenal Glands

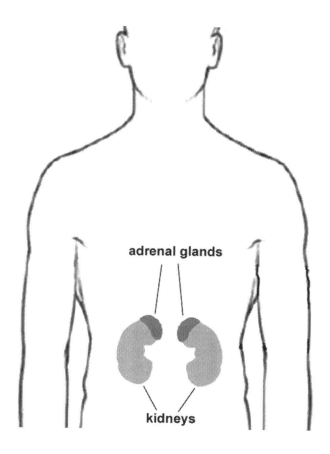

adrenal glands

kidneys

The adrenal glands are on top of the kidneys. They have a core, an inner part, called the medulla (the same term used for the lowest third of the brain stem), and a surrounding surface called a cortex (the same term used for the surface structures of the brain itself). The core produces the hormones epinephrine and norepinephrine, also called adrenaline and noradrenaline. These are chemicals released and active in response to *acute stress*. The cortex, or surface of the adrenal glands, produces cortisol or glucocorticoids, *long-term stress* chemicals, and also aldosterone, a hormone that helps regulate kidney function, and testosterone, a sex hormone with other functions as well.

H-P-A Axis (Hypothalamus-Pituitary-Adrenal Axis)

H-P-A AXIS (Hypothalamus-Pituitary-Adrenal Axis)

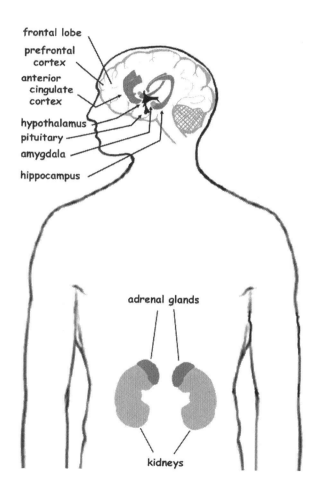

There are biochemical messages that travel from the hypothalamus to the pituitary gland and then, by means of the vascular/hormone system, down to the adrenal glands. The adrenal glands in turn send messages back to the brain. This is a brain/body connection. The brain and body are not separate. They never have been separate. Any separation is totally imaginary and arbitrary. Whenever the brain experiences something, so does the body. Whenever the body experiences something, so does the brain.

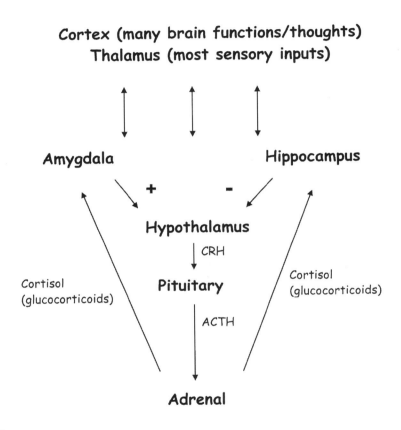

Notes:
- Hypothalamus-Pituitary-Adrenal is called HPA axis.
- All the structures except the adrenal glands are parts of the brain. The adrenal glands are on top of the kidneys.
- + means increased/exciting message activity
- - means decreased/calming message activity
- CRH is corticotrophin releasing hormone
- ACTH is adrenocorticotropic hormone
- Glucocorticoid is long-term stress chemical

Stimulation of the brain/body by means of pain or stress, or thoughts, feelings, and behaviors associated with pain or stress, activates the amygdala and hippocampus, as well as other brain parts. These in turn transmit messages through the brain to stimulate the hypothalamus. The hypothalamus then releases chemicals called ***corticotropin releasing hormone (CRH)*** which in turn stimulate the pituitary gland. The anterior or front part of the pituitary gland releases a chemical called ***adrenocorticotropic hormone (ACTH)*** which travels into and through the blood throughout the body and to the adrenal glands. The adrenal glands then secrete glucocorticoids, cortisone, steroids that travel through the blood back up to the brain and re-stimulate the amygdala and hippocampus to do it some more. This is a clear and obvious example of the brain/body connection. The ***Hypothalamus-Pituitary-Adrenal*** connection is called ***the H-P-A axis.*** The H-P-A axis is one very important network of brain/body connection. It seems to be key in understanding much of the emotional dysregulation and the difficulties with cognition when the person is struggling with long-term pain.

Normally there is a nice balance between the effects of the amygdala, with its intense emotional content, and the hippocampus, with its reasoning mechanisms. The messages from the hippocampus tend to calm the flow of messages from the amygdala and its intense emotional activity. This balance between the amygdala (emotion) and the hippocampus (logic and reason) keeps the flow of messages and chemicals more stable and useful for our daily lives. Our emotions may be calmed by our thinking, or our emotions may be intensified by our thinking. Our thinking is significantly influenced by our emotional experiences.

When the amygdala is stimulated by the glucocorticoid from the adrenal glands, it gets all excited and starts sending more stimulating messages to the hypothalamus, thus prompting more of the HPA axis involvement. When there is a significant amount of long-term stress, the long-term stress chemical glucocorticoid causes significant stimulation of the amygdala. The amygdala then becomes hypersensitive to this chemical. In a way, it seems to thrive on the stimulation and the amygdala becomes hyperactive, causing continued and excessive output of electro-chemical activity. This stimulates the hypothalamus again, which in turn stimulates the pituitary gland, which again stimulates the adrenal glands, which in turn sends out more glucocorticoid. This long-term stress chemical then travels through the blood stream and back to the amygdala, stimulating it to send more of its messages. This may be the underlying neuro-bio-chemical foundation of various anxiety and mood disorders. The problems become circular in that the person starts to become anxious about being anxious, and depressed about being depressed. Pain interrupts sleep and lack of sleep worsens pain. It worsens as time progresses.

The amygdala can be calmed by many approaches and many brain parts and networks can be involved in this process. One of the brain parts that can have a calming influence on the amygdala is the hippocampus. Glucocorticoid goes to both the amygdala and the hippocampus. The right amount of glucocorticoid to the hippocampus can stimulate the activity of the hippocampus which might calm and dampen, to a degree, the hyperactivity of the amygdala. But it has to be the right amount. Too little is not good, and too much is not good.

The Goldilocks Experience

In 1837, the British author and poet, Robert Southey, wrote the story of *Goldilocks and the Three Bears*. He tells of Goldilocks sampling the various items in the bear house and experiencing the beds as being too soft, too hard, or just right, or the porridge being too cold, too hot, or just right. Similarly, glucocorticoid levels need to be just right in order for us to function normally.

Too little can be problematic. The hippocampus needs a certain level of glucocorticoid stimulation in order to function well. We need some level of stressful stimulation to think and focus clearly. A person might plan out the details of a talk or presentation ahead of time in order to be prepared and ready. A person might study in advance of a test and be truly ready to do well. A little bit of stress, or just the right amount of stress, can be helpful. If the person comes into the situation too relaxed, without preparation, planning, effort, and organization, he or she might not do well.

Too much glucocorticoid excreted from the adrenal glands and stimulating the hippocampus might be disruptive to the thinking and memory processes. Too much glucocorticoid stimulating the hippocampus can lead to disruptions in the connections and functions of the cells of the hippocampus. Too much stress might result in "stage fright" or "test anxiety."

If the long-term stress is severe enough, it may also result in actual dying off of some cells of the hippocampus, thus making the hippocampus somewhat smaller, or "hippocampal atrophy." This of course lessens the balancing or moderating effect of the hippocampus on the amygdala and the H-P-A axis and thus the amygdala and its emotional memories and experiences becomes excessively strong and less modulated by the calming effects of the logical, reasonable, practical, sensible, and level headed hippocampus.

The hippocampus, which is more involved in episodic memory, memory of the details of a specific episode or occurrence rather than the emotions of the experience, might not work as well when there is too much glucocorticoid stimulating the hippocampus. The thinking, reasoning, calming, decision making, and clear memory and judgment aspects of the situation or experience might not work as well when there is too much glucocorticoid exciting the amygdala and dampening the hippocampus.

You may not be able to remember why you went into a room, where you put your car keys, or worse yet, where you parked your car. You may have high anxiety. You may rarely feel calm. You may have problems with memory, judgment, decision-making, learning new material, and long-term memory consolidation and retrieval. You may have trouble making decisions and plans about your future because the emotional experience is too intense. The practical, reasoning abilities might be dimmed and dulled and inadequate to the tasks.

Just the right amount of glucocorticoid is what one would hope for. This usually occurs normally by itself. This is called **homeostasis**. This is an ongoing dance or choreographed process involving the H-P-A axis and other mind/body connections that keep everything stable and comfortable. It occurs naturally, consistently, and subconsciously, unless there is injury to the brain, or unless we develop habits of emotion, behavior, and thought that disrupt the choreography.

Balance Is best. Better and stronger connections between neurons can occur everywhere in the nervous system. Weakening of connections can also occur. Understanding that these processes occur can help one to utilize techniques and procedures for self-enhancing benefits rather than self-defeating behaviors. Either way, neurons and their connections change constantly.

Most of this brain/body activity is automatic or subconscious. It is constantly happening without our full awareness. However, with conscious practice, many things can be changed. Think of Pavlov's "classical conditioning" experiments with dogs. Dogs normally salivate when they are presented with meat. We presume they are also ready and hungry and want to eat the meat. When they hear a bell just before they are presented with the meat, and this is done repetitively, they very quickly learn to salivate when they hear the bell. You can see that this salivation is an automatic, autonomic response to a stimulus. It is not done on purpose. It is a brain/body subconscious automatic response. This is what occurs when one pairs a stimulus like a bell just before giving the meat to the dogs. Similar things happen to us humans.

The meat is called the ***unconditioned stimulus***, because it doesn't require any training to elicit the response of salivating. The bell is called the ***conditioned stimulus***, because it does require training and conditioning in order to elicit the response of salivating. Salivation is the response. It is tied to the unconditioned stimulus, the meat; and with training, it is eventually tied to the conditioned stimulus, the bell. Responses are not simply physiologic like salivation. They can also be thoughts and feelings. The hunger the animal feels as it desires to eat meat is also a response. There are many responses in the brain/body to the conditioned and unconditioned stimuli. Salivation, because it was more observable, is the response that Pavlov paid attention to.

This might be similar to the experience of a patient who was injured at his place of employment and experienced a great deal of pain, suffering, and then a sense of injustice in the whole situation. The response of feeling fear or anger is tied to the unconditioned stimulus of feeling pain. The response of feeling fear or anger can also become tied to the conditioned stimulus. The conditioned stimulus is the learned phenomenon. One can learn to feel anger and pain even at the sight or thought of his place of work where he was injured or treated poorly. Just thinking about his work can bring about the feelings of anger, fear, the sense of injustice, and the physical experience of muscle tightness and pain. So even a thought can be a stimulus and lead to feelings and responses. A response in turn can become another stimulus. This can be cyclical.

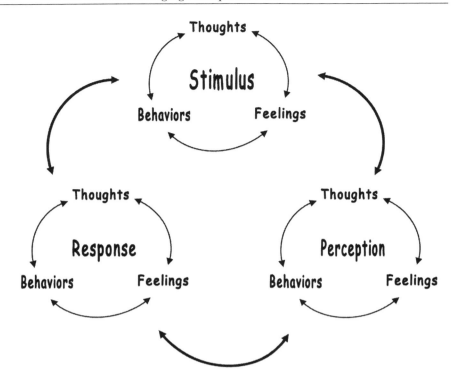

The thought of the specific work setting has become a conditioned stimulus for the response and feelings of pain, anger, fear, and sense of injustice. Autonomic and peripheral responses include increased blood pressure and pulse, sweating, and muscle tightness. Centrally the pain, anger, anxiety, and suffering are experienced. Again, one thing leads to another and the proverbial vicious cycle is perpetuated.

A patient described going on a driving vacation. He felt more calm and relaxed once he got fifty miles away from his usual setting. His usual setting was, in his perception, his usual stressful workplace. He also described becoming very tense and having an increase in pain when returning home from vacation. He began to feel miserable when he was only fifty miles away from home. This is an example of thought being a stimulus that causes the response of feeling miserable. Feeling miserable can in turn be a stimulus for thinking worse thoughts.

Another patient, an injured employee at a different company, described the voice and words of his employer on the telephone when he was finally told he could return to work. His employer said that he would be making $2 less per hour. The patient's muscles became very tight around his neck and a headache came on almost immediately. In biological terms, his amygdala was stimulated and sent messages to his pons, which in turn sent messages to his sympathetic nervous system, and then to the muscles around his neck and head.

The mind/body is connected. The brain/body is connected. They cannot be separated. What the body feels, the brain experiences. What the brain does affects the body. Can our thought processes and emotional response to our experiences make us worse or better?

Anterior Cingulate Cortex (ACC)

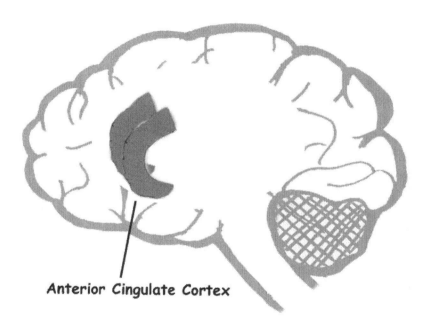

Anterior Cingulate Cortex

There are many other areas of the brain that experience pain and its associated emotional content. Neural messages from the body are transmitted to all these areas. Neural messages, including messages from painful stimuli, go to the somatosensory cortex to tell us where in the corresponding area of the body the pain is actually and specifically being felt. When neural messages go to the emotionally sensitive and responsive areas, pain becomes more than pain. It can become suffering. The *anterior cingulate cortex (ACC)* is one of brain's structures that can experience and, interestingly, amplify the painful message, resulting in suffering. Electrical stimulation of the anterior cingulate cortex in rats has lessened pain responses associated with mechanical allodynia. Is it possible that the thoughts of a human being could be used to stimulate the anterior cingulate cortex in various ways to worsen or lessen pain at will?

The anterior cingulate cortex is a key region in the brain for processing pain. It lights up in response to pain anywhere in the body. However, the anterior cingulate cortex lights up for many other reasons as well. If the anterior cingulate cortex is stimulated by a small electrical impulse, without any painful stimulus, the person will feel a distressed, uncomfortable mood.

The anterior cingulate cortex is an emotional alarm system. It draws the brain's attention to distressing or unexpected changes in the environment. This is for safety and survival. It then sends messages to other parts of the nervous system and body to bring about appropriate responses for safety, escape, freezing in place, fight, flight, problem solving, and so on.

Hypnosis to block out pain actually blocks out the responses in the anterior cingulate cortex, but not the somatosensory cortex. A patient going through a low back surgery with no anesthesia, using hypnosis instead, interpreted the sensation of the scalpel as a cold ice cube running down the middle of the low back. The person interpreted the dripping of blood across the skin as the ice cube melting. The person did not feel the pain as expected and stated that she did not really feel pain. Certain thoughts that this person created in other brain parts calmed the anterior cingulate cortex.

The opposite experience can also occur. If a person has been conditioned to expect sharp pain, but in reality is stimulated with something non-painful, like a warm touch, the anterior cingulate cortex reacts as though it were a painful stimulus. The anterior cingulate cortex helps one learn and remember important things about the painful experience. But it is not always accurate.

Rats with damage to the anterior cingulate cortex still react to pain in the foot by flinching or licking the foot, but they do not learn to avoid the painful stimulus. The anterior cingulate cortex, when working well, helps the rats learn and remember something very important about certain experiences. Without this part of the brain working well the rat may not learn and remember to avoid the painful stimulus.

So what might all this mean to humans? What happens when the anterior cingulate cortex is too active or not working well enough? How does the anterior cingulate cortex develop normally? What if it develops abnormally? Can a person change and improve the function of the anterior cingulate cortex later in life, and can this make a difference in the painful experience?

The cingulate cortex is large and deep within the brain. The anterior cingulate cortex is the front part of the cingulate cortex, a component of the limbic system. Deep within the frontal lobes, the anterior cingulate cortex, along with other brain parts and networks, is responsible to a degree for mood and impulse control. One of the specific functions of the anterior cingulate cortex is to help shift attention from one thing to another. For example, it lights up when a mother hears a baby's cry.

Normally, we are constantly shifting attention from one thing to the other all day long and during the night as well. Sometimes the shifting mechanisms can "get stuck." *Obsessive compulsive disorder (OCD)* may be an example of this. The person says something like, "I keep having these anxious thoughts..." They are intrusive, repetitive thoughts. Then the person might say something like, "I do these specific things to relieve the thoughts and bad feelings." These behaviors become ritualistic activities to relieve the tension or anxiety associated with the thoughts. Then the person feels some sense of relief after performing the behavior.

The classic example, of course, is the person who thinks and feels that his hands are dirty and covered with germs. He is constantly driven to wash them, over and over, all day, until they are red and raw. Obsessive thoughts and terrible anxious feelings are partly relieved by the compulsive behavior. The person washes his hands too much, which hurts the hands, but he feels better emotionally, with lessened anxiety, at least temporarily.

This process and pattern can become a deeply and repetitively ingrained, neuron-bio-electro-chemical pathway or pattern in the networks of the brain, spinal cord, and body. One thing leads to another, and leads to another. This is done over and over until it is very difficult to actually do anything differently than the process that the nervous system and body is used to. It becomes very difficult to change the behavior or pattern.

The pain path can be very similar. The person is hurt at work. Thus the person's job/workplace and pain/injury become connected deeply in their thoughts, feelings, and brain/body, even on a subconscious level. The experience of pain is an unconditioned stimulus. Remember that unconditioned means that the person does not have to learn about it. It just happens naturally, like feeling pain when stuck with a needle. This is a biological function that most of us are born with and do not need any learning to experience.

The painful stimulus results in a number of understandable and expected responses. These include neurobiological, biochemical, and physiological experiences such as anxiety, depression, and muscle tightness. All of these responses can lead to a worsening and continuation of the painful experience.

There are also a number of behavioral responses such as the pain behaviors of grimacing, limping, guarding, and avoidance of activities that might be done to lessen the painful experience but sometimes can also lead to a more painful experience. Compensating one part of the body with another part of the body can lead to pain in the compensating part. Behavioral responses might also include the use of drugs and other alternative states. All of these responses can lead to feeling somewhat better with respect to the particular painful experience. Feeling somewhat better, however, can lead to return to work, thoughts of return to work, or return to other activities that, in turn, can worsen the pain at the time.

For some people, return to work, thoughts of return to work, and the site of the work place become a conditioned stimulus. This means that there is learning that occurs. The anterior cingulate cortex is working. The person was not born with anxiety about return to work. The person learned this because of the experience with pain as related to the work experience. This can be physical pain and/or emotional pain. The stimulus can bring about the neurobiological, biochemical, and physiological experiences such as anxiety and its physical symptoms and other behavioral responses.

Hamster mothers with injury to the anterior cingulate cortex no longer take steps to keep their pups near, and infant squirrel monkeys with damage to the anterior cingulate cortex no longer cry when separated from their mothers. How might this relate to humans? A person in too much pain or on too much pain medication may have somewhat less motivation to care appropriately or thoroughly for their children or others close to them. Normal functioning of the anterior cingulate cortex might keep one close and interested and drawn to their loved ones.

The anterior cingulate cortex is more active when the person is reporting distress associated with social exclusion or rejection. Imagine what it was like in your youth, or might have been like, to be chosen last in sporting events and activities. This may be similar to when the person is experiencing pain, at least emotionally, and in how the anterior cingulate cortex is stimulated and responds. It is emotionally painful to experience social rejection and exclusion, like shunning in some religious cultures or organizations, or perceived invalidation in the worker's compensation or medical system. This occurs when the person is treated as though the medical problem is imaginary or psychological. This experience can literally be painful. Rejection hurts, literally. "Sticks and stones will break my bones, but names will never hurt me." Not true.

The anterior cingulate cortex is more active when the person is reporting distress associated with social exclusion or rejection.

Painful messages and visual, auditory, and cognitive inputs go to the amygdala, the anterior cingulate cortex, and many other brain nuclei and networks caught up and implicated in the emotional content of the pain and the meaning of the painful experience in the person's life. Even just thinking about a situation can stimulate the amygdala to sense and transmit the anxious, fearful, painful messages to the other brain parts and down into the body. Repetitively thinking in negative terms about a particular situation, or allowing yourself to repetitively feel certain emotions, will strengthen those processes, neural pathways, and brain/body connections. Repetitively thinking and behaving in self-defeating ways will strengthen pathways in the nervous system and the brain/body connections that you probably don't want to strengthen. You may have to practice something else. Do you want to practice making things worse, or practice making things better?

Repetitively thinking and behaving in self-defeating ways will strengthen pathways in the nervous system and the brain/body connections that you probably don't want to strengthen.

How To Make Some Things Better

There are many things that can help make the hippocampus, frontal lobe, and other brain networks work better. There are many ways to calm the emotional dysregulation of the amygdala, the anterior cingulate cortex, and other emotionally charged limbic networks.

One of the things that may stimulate the hippocampus to work better and calm the amygdala is interpersonal therapy. When a person visits with the psychologist and uses cognitive behavioral techniques, or other psychological techniques, to gain a sense of control over the emotions, the person feels better. The psychologist might say something like, "Let's think about this together, and let's come up with a plan together to solve this problem. Let's make a list of the pros and cons and let's prioritize these issues." This type of counseling and interpersonal therapy stimulates the hippocampus to work better. It can facilitate stronger connections between the neurons of the hippocampus. It can also result in hippocampal neurogenesis, or the creation of new neurons in the hippocampus. Interpersonal therapy can make the hippocampus work better. The person can develop a larger and more active hippocampus. This creation of new cells can occur throughout our entire lives.

The anterior cingulate cortex is calmed by social support, caring, love, respect, and understanding. The subconscious connection between the patient and a caring therapist or between the patient and other understanding and validating people can be very calming and comforting. Patients can be asked many years after the three week residential pain management program, "What was the best part of the program for you?" They will answer, "The other patients, the support from the other patients, and the caring staff." We all need love and support. After the pain program, one of the most important factors that seems to facilitate long-term success with respect to return to life, and even decreased pain, is social support. One might imagine that the anterior cingulate cortex "feels good" when there is love and support. More realistically, calming of the anterior cingulate cortex must stimulate associated networks including the nucleus accumbens and its dopamine and pleasure pathways and experiences.

Another important factor in continued and long-term healing seems to be daily scheduled activity and structure in daily life. Structured daily activity after the pain program is extremely important. Structure in daily activity must somehow stimulate the frontal lobe and the hippocampus and result in calming of the amygdala and the anterior cingulate cortex.

Of interest is the fact that the right ventral pre-frontal cortex regulates distress of social exclusion by disrupting anterior cingulate cortex activity. This is a good thing. The right ventral pre-frontal cortex also lights up in social exclusionary situations, but its ability to contemplate, reason, think ahead and plan can help calm down the emotionally distressed anterior cingulate cortex.

One can practice and learn to think about reasonable and practical approaches to difficulties. One can learn and practice daily active structure in one's life. This is usually similar to what was going on before pain came onboard. Thinking clearly is often quite different than what is going on in one's life after pain comes onboard. One can lessen the emotional impact of painful situations to a degree, by focusing on, strengthening, and using the more logical, reasonable mindset. This does not mean that people are not reasonable, or that emotions are bad or inappropriate, but sometimes powerful emotions and the emotional content of the painful experience can disrupt logical, reasonable thinking and functioning. On the other hand, the emotionally painful content and experience can be modulated or calmed by reasonable thinking and structured behavior. We can change much of the chemistry of the chronic pain cycle by calming the emotionally charged amygdala and anterior cingulate cortex.

Dr. Muhammad Yunus' Unifying Theory

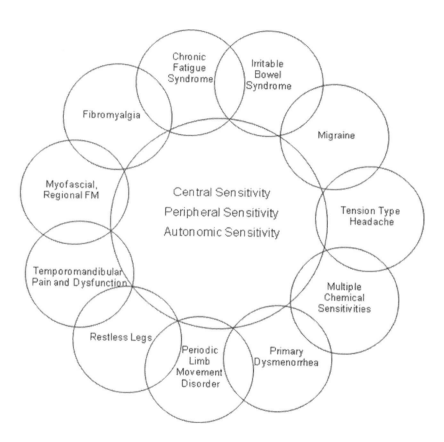

Chronic Fatigue Syndrome

Irritable Bowel Syndrome

Fibromyalgia

Migraine

Myofascial, Regional FM

Central Sensitivity
Peripheral Sensitivity
Autonomic Sensitivity

Tension Type Headache

Temporomandibular Pain and Dysfunction

Multiple Chemical Sensitivities

Restless Legs

Periodic Limb Movement Disorder

Primary Dysmenorrhea

Central Sensitivity Syndrome

This term was coined by Dr. Muhammad Yunus in 1984 to describe the relationship and unifying concept among these various conditions. There are many conditions which seem to be related or connected to each other in some way. Dr. Yunus called this unifying concept *The Central Sensitivity Syndrome (CSS)*. He did not include peripheral or autonomic involvement. It has also been called *Central Neuroendocrine Dysregulation*. It implies that the central nervous system and the endocrine systems are involved in the process or phenomenon. It also implies that these systems become very sensitive or abnormally hypersensitive and hyperreactive to various stimuli.

In reality it seems that the hypersensitivity and hyperreactivity involve more than just the central nervous system. Many of these conditions listed might be related to central hypersensitivity, but also to peripheral and/or autonomic hypersensitivity. The hypersensitivity may be present in the periphery, the skin, muscles, internal organs, and the hyperreactive responses may include the autonomic/sympathetic nervous system as well.

Often when a patient with fibromyalgia is shown this picture of circles and this concept, the person is shocked at the fact that she or he has several, if not all, of the conditions at the same time. Does the person really have eight or ten different diseases or conditions? Probably not. Does the person have one condition which manifests in various ways? Probably. This one condition might be the hypersensitivity and hyperactivity of the various parts of the nervous system.

In addition to the disorders listed by Dr. Yunus, there may be many other disorders that somehow involve these same hypersensitive and hyperreactive phenomena. There may also be many other factors that aggravate or perpetuate these various conditions. There may be many factors that influence the perceptions and responses of each individual person. The following diagram hypothesizes (by this author) the relationship or association of many other conditions under the unifying concept of the hypersensitive and hyperreactive nervous system.

Other Conditions

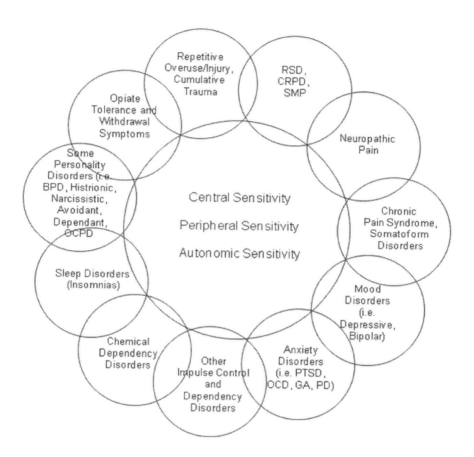

See Glossary for further details.

If you cause pain in a mouse's paw for a few hours the mouse will display or demonstrate pain behaviors. It won't step on the paw normally. It will limp. It won't drink its sugar water or have sex as probably nothing is very pleasurable. It won't or can't sleep. Other mice in the cage end up on the other side of the cage, probably because the mouse is driving them away, although we cannot ask the little guy if he was being grumpy and irritable and driving all his friends and relatives away. We can't ask the mouse if he feels depressed or anxious or what his pain level is, but the mouse does make vocalizations, probably crying or whining or groaning. This seems very much like what a person experiences, or at least how a person behaves when struggling with pain.

When the painful stimulus is removed completely, the mouse no longer demonstrates any pain behaviors. The pain behaviors go away. As far as we can tell, it does not hurt any more. This is what we would expect and hope for when surgery or some other medical procedure is performed to fix a medical problem in a person as well.

If the painful stimulus is continued in the mouse paw for several weeks, a different picture presents after the stimulus is removed. The painful behaviors do not go away. The mouse still hurts even though the paw is fixed. This is very much like a human being who has gone through surgery to fix something that has been there a long time, but the pain still persists or continues. Could there be something else going on in the mouse or the human being that is more complex than simply the pain and pathology in the paw or body part?

A mouse only lives for two years or so, so a painful experience lasting several weeks for the mouse may be like "chronic pain" for a human being. Chronic pain or long-term pain causes changes in various parts and cells of the brain, the spinal cord, the peripheral nervous system, and autonomic nervous system of the mouse and probably the human being as well. We can dissect the mouse, or many mice, to find out this type of information but we cannot do this so easily with human beings. There are changes in the nervous system of the mouse, and there are probably changes in the nervous system of the human being, when pain is experienced for a long time. These changes may be related to some of the long-term or persistent pain that people experience in spite of the medical treatment.

The changes that occur in the central nervous system, the peripheral nervous system, and the autonomic nervous system may not necessarily be permanent. Researchers are trying to find ways to change the cells, brain, spinal cord, or other brain/body functions to lessen the pain. They are trying to find ways to return things back to normal or to change things somehow so that pain will not persist after the painful stimulus has been removed.

Central sensitivity, peripheral sensitivity, and autonomic sensitivity syndromes can occur when the nervous system becomes oversensitive or hypersensitive to various types of stimuli. A person might be hypersensitive to various stimuli in the psychobiological realm as well. These might include phobias, thoughts, or sensitivity to any stimuli that make a person feel afraid or anxious. It is not clearly understood how or why this process occurs in some cases and not in others. Genetic predispositions, early environmental influences, ongoing life experiences, physiologic and biochemical processes, and incalculable other factors account for individual differences of human beings.

Jack, a thirty year old man, was involved in an automobile accident and nine months later needed low back surgery. He was seen in consultation for the ongoing pain five months post-surgery. He was on high dose opioids [1], weaned off, and returned to normal life activities. However, he described how he thought the sympathetic nervous system was extremely sensitive for many months

---

1   (the equivalent of 280 mg of Oxycodone daily. This is equivalent to fifty-six Percocet tablets every day (without the Tylenol). It still was not working very well to lessen pain or improve function. He gradually weaned down to 135 mg of Oxycodone, about twenty-seven Percocet per day, with difficulty and some ups and downs, not following the weaning schedule exactly. Eventually we decided to use Suboxone. He used 2/0.5 mg tablets (buprenorphine 2 mg, and nalaxone 0.5 mg) four tablets, two times per day. This worked dramatically well to lessen withdrawal symptoms and help him stay off the opioids. He was able to go back to work at a job that was not so physically demanding. He still felt pain, but less so. Any problems he was having with withdrawal symptoms went away completely. He gradually weaned off the Suboxone over a two month time period.)

during this whole situation. He said, "I would take a hot shower and get goosebumps. I felt anxious constantly. I blushed easily. My legs jerked and twitched when something irritated my skin as I was trying to fall asleep at night." The simplest stimulation to the skin caused obvious and significant movement and sympathetic responses. All of this did settle down and change over time.

A person can not only be hypersensitive to various external stimuli, but also to internal stimuli like thoughts and emotions. There are many people who tend to give "110 percent" effort in their job situation. They could probably wear a tee shirt that says, "Always remember, your job is more important than you are." There is a condition called repetitive over use syndrome or cumulative trauma disorder where a person begins feeling pain when doing a repetitive job activity. If the person does not stop or be careful in the job setting, he or she could be injured significantly. The person might keep working hard, ignoring the problem, hoping the problem will work itself out and go away, but instead the pain becomes worse and worse. Over time, it doesn't require as much stimulation to cause the more severe pain. It hurts when doing almost nothing, and hurts worse when doing more strenuous activities. The person feels the pain with the slightest stimulation. If the problem is in the arms and hands, the pain may be felt when doing something as simple as writing, typing, trying to play cards, or doing simple personal hygiene.

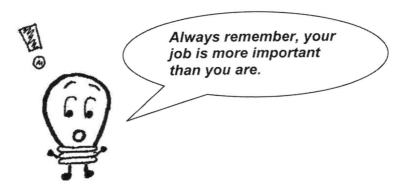

Always remember, your job is more important than you are.

In addition to this physical injury this same person might experience an internal underlying sense of anxiety. This might be a fairly consistent, low grade, and long lasting underlying discomfort, or it could be a sudden, intense, short term episode of anxiety. Symptoms might include apprehension, fearfulness, terror, a sense of impending doom, fear of going crazy, or fear of losing control. There can be symptoms such as shortness of breath, palpitations, chest pain or discomfort, choking, or smothering sensations. A person might experience it as an almost irresistible desire to change something or escape. The person might have a specific phobia, and when exposed to the object or situation, might experience a tremendous drive to get away from it. The person becomes hypersensitive to this particular stimulus. The person becomes hyperreactive as well, and then experiences relief when he or she gets away from the stimulus. The relief becomes a positive reinforcer for the hyperreactive, withdrawal behavior, a learned behavior and pattern. This learned behavior and pattern becomes consistent, strong, almost obsessive, compulsive, and hard to change.

Jerry, an attorney on the Boston Legal television show, has *Asperger's*, according to the show. One of the descriptive characteristics of this condition is an obsessive quality to his interest in only one thing in life. This might even be to the detriment of interest in other things. Jerry's interest is the law. He has an encyclopedic knowledge of the Massachusetts legal code. But he is handicapped in his ability to switch his thoughts, feelings, and behaviors to other things. He is stuck in the law. He might not know how to survive when traveling to another country or how to enjoy ice fishing or how to raise a child. This is not to say that other people with this condition cannot function and be successful in many things. It is just that Jerry is presented this way in the program.

Pain, in general, may be a survival mechanism, but it can also be detrimental to our lives. We pay attention. We focus. We obsess, even to the detriment of involvement in other activities and people and purposes. This seems to be normal with respect to pain. But it is very difficult to change the focus when experiencing pain.

Maybe we all have obsessions and compulsions to a degree, but not to the point of pathology where we cannot be interested, involved, or successful in other things. People have hobbies and interests, such as hunting, fishing, chess, collecting, history, playing mandolin. Usually we can change, adapt, and focus attention and interest from one thing to another without too much difficulty. But when in pain it is hard to think of anything else.

What makes a person be able to change focus? What makes things interesting to one person and boring to another? For example, what makes it easy for one person to remember all the facts concerning England's Henry VIII stories, his wives, his children, and all the relationships? A person once told me that her interest in the Henry VIII stories and history was because of her interest and thoughts about power. Another person might be interested because of the stories of beheadings. Another might be interested in the political history of the time.

Someone might be very interested in biology, maybe obsessively so, and try to explain things to other people only in biological terms. The other people may tune out, stare with glossy eyes into the distance, and feel lost and bored, because they may not have this same interest.

Pain and pleasure draw our interest and attention. They must somehow stimulate attention networks and pathways in the brain. Pain and pleasure somehow promote and facilitate desire for repetition of particular activities. In general, this is to avoid the pain, or to repeat the pleasure experience.

Pain stimulates pathways and networks that facilitate self-protection. Can pain, physical and emotional, also stimulate pathways and networks that facilitate protection of loved ones? What is happening in the brain of a parent whose daughter moves far away to a place where there are relationship and safety problems? Why does that parent think and obsess about the daughter and the situation? It is not pleasurable. Indeed, we can obsess about something that is pleasurable, but also about things that are not pleasurable. When we obsess we are practicing and strengthening particular biochemical and neurological pathways. When was obsess and then behave in compulsive ways we are further strengthening particular biochemical and neurological pathways.

Why do we think and talk with other people about something we are obsessing about? We talk and talk and talk with ourselves and others. Will it help find solutions? Is the talking itself calming somehow? Does thinking or talking calm down the free-floating anxiety as we obsess about something that is not pleasurable or crave something that is pleasurable? Are words and thoughts more controlled and comforting than the anxiety? Are the feelings the obsessions? Are the thoughts and words the compulsions? Does the person become hypersensitive and hyperreactive to these various internal stimuli? Are some biochemical and neurological pathways strengthened and others changed? Is this what happens in treatment programs for various dependencies?

Dependency and impulse control disorders are very complex. They involve obsessions and compulsions. The person obsesses about their cravings and feelings, then responds with the compulsive behavior such as drink alcohol, ingest pills, breath in smoke, or gamble. The person may experience many uncomfortable cognitive, emotional, behavioral, and physiological symptoms. A pattern of repeated self-administration to soothe and comfort can result eventually in tolerance, or needing more and more to do the same job. Trying to break the well developed pattern of repeated self-administration to soothe and comfort can result in withdrawal symptoms.

The Diagnostic and Statistical Manual, DSM-IV-TR, describes a great deal of information about various drugs and chemicals and their effects on the brain/body. It does not describe what happens in the brain/body of the person; the thoughts, feelings, and behaviors associated with the drive, attraction, and compulsion to use or participate in the particular activity.

A person practices or repetitively performs a particular behavior and experiences positive reinforcement, pleasure or relief of discomfort. The desire to do the behavior or activity or use the drug becomes stronger and stronger. This again is called sensitization. Some examples might include the positive reinforcement of catching a fish when fishing, or getting a strike when bowling. Positive reinforcement is experienced when hitting a very good shot while golfing, or hearing the clanging of the coins when hitting a jackpot while gambling. Positive reinforcement is experienced when feeling pleasure with sex, being able to place one card on another when playing spider solitaire, or getting a high when drinking alcohol.

Sensitization is essentially the opposite of habituation. Both are learned. With repetitive exposure to a particular stimulus, the person or animal becomes either more sensitive and responsive (sensitization), or less sensitive and responsive (habituation). A person might be very sensitive to the smell of new paint in a house, but then fairly quickly might habituate and not even smell the paint anymore.

Remember the bears in Yellowstone that habituated to people and cars? They don't run away so quickly and basically respond less to the presence of people or passing cars. Why a person sometimes develops habituation versus sensitization is unclear. A person may become habituated to one thing, like medications or opioids, and sensitized to another, like pain, all at the same time.

Tolerance to a medication or drug may be like habituation in that the person becomes less sensitive to the effects of the medication. The person needs more and more of the chemical or the particular stimulus to do the same job. This is a very common problem with opioid use over the long run.

Withdrawal symptoms, in a way, are more like being hypersensitive to the decreased amount of the medication, drug, or other stimulus. Withdrawal symptoms shout out loudly at first but then gradually quiet down and burn out. The person may actually be hypersensitive for a while to his or her own symptoms associated with lessened use of the medication, drug, or other stimulus. The person may then habituate to the new medication level.

Withdrawal symptoms associated with controlled substance discontinuation vary for many reasons. The specific drug, the quantity, the frequency of use, the length of time the medication was taken, and the individual person are all important factors. Withdrawal symptoms are basically opposite of the drug effect.

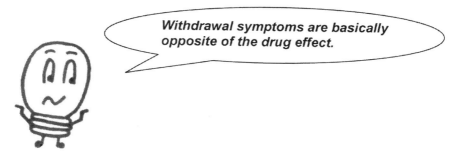

Withdrawal symptoms are basically opposite of the drug effect.

Opioid (narcotic) withdrawal symptoms *may* include: increased pain, craving, restlessness, anxiety, sweating, yawning, irritability, increased sensitivity, nasal congestion, cramping, muscle twitching/tremor, depression, anxiety, emotional lability, fever, increased blood pressure, increased pulse rate, gooseflesh skin (goosebumps), insomnia, coughing, nausea, vomiting, diarrhea, and dilated pupils. Benzodiazepines are also controlled substances. Their withdrawal symptoms *may* include: anxiety, irritability, hallucinations, muscle aches, twitching, depression, emotional lability, sleep disturbance, panic, increased sensitivity to light and sound, tremors, seizures, and constricted pupils. Even the abrupt discontinuation of anti-depressants can result in flu-like symptoms, nausea, insomnia, hyper-arousal, imbalance, and sensory disturbances.

Cecilia, a forty year old woman with fibromyalgia, wanted to get off opioids. She had been using ten Vicodin per day for six years. She felt that she was using the medication just to feel relatively normal, to get up to a normal baseline physically and psychologically. She weaned off slowly and successfully. She stated that the pain felt worse each time she lowered the dose of the medication, but then eventually this increase in pain settled down. Her nervous system was sensitized to the pain. She stated, referring to being on the medication versus being off the medication, "It was like walking in water, or on top of the water, versus walking finally on solid ground. Like being stable and no longer having a feeling as though sinking all the time." She was seen in follow-up several months later. She had not experienced much in the way of withdrawal symptoms. She stated that her pain, in the end, was really no worse than when on the medication. She stated, "I will never go back on those again." We know that she might someday for some acute problem, surgery, dental procedure, broken limb, or whatever, but this was her experience, perspective, and comments at the time. She had become tolerant to the medication. She had habituated to the medication. It was really not doing much in terms of pain relief. It was affecting her sense of stability, although she did not recognize this while on the medication. She needed to get off it and spend some time in that state of being to really recognize the difference.

Della, a forty year old woman with fibromyalgia, described her experience when accidentally running out of medications four days early. She was very tearful, anxious, and in significant pain. The medications included Klonopin (a benzodiazepine, anti-anxiety medication), Tripleptal (anti-seizure and sometimes helpful for certain types of nerve pain), Cymbalta (anti-depressant and sometimes helpful for certain types of nerve pain), Ultram (non-narcotic analgesic), Norflex (muscle relaxer), and Nortriptyline (anti-depressant, sometimes helpful for certain types of nerve pain and usually helpful for sleep)[2]. She described withdrawal and dis-

---

2   Actual doses of the medications were as follows: Klonopin 0.5 mg, 15–30 per month, Tripleptal 150 mg three times per day, Cymbalta 90 mg per day, Ultram 50 mg three times per day, Norflex 100 mg twice daily, and Nortriptyline 50 mg at bed time.

continuation syndrome, including flu-like symptoms, nausea and vomiting, emotional lability, trembling, sweating, and tingling all over. She felt extremely anxious and tense, "increased nerve pain" in her limbs, depressed, irritable, confusion, and could not sleep. She stated that it was too difficult to handle. She was angry and irritable with family members. She was tearful, on edge, and could hardly function at work. She stated that work was more stressful anyway with the poor economy, but the stress of being off medications made everything worse as well. The CNS (central nervous system), PNS (peripheral nervous system), and ANS (autonomic nervous system) were all being affected by these medications and were all hypersensitive and hyperreactive when off these medications.

Antonio was a forty-four year Hispanic gentleman with a ten year history of back and leg pain associated with a worker's compensation injury. During the years after the injury, and prior to a three week pain program, he also had three back surgeries, one with the complication of infection. He had a three decade history of chemical dependency and for years before the pain program was on about 200 mg of Oxycontin daily (about forty Percocet per day, without the Tylenol). He worked very hard on a weaning plan and eventually switched to Suboxone and worked on weaning off this. He stated near the end of the weaning process, "I am weaning off Suboxone. Today is my last day. When I was down to one pill per day, I started feeling cravings for crack. I haven't felt this in seven years." He said that, "Withdrawal feels like restless leg syndrome on crack," totally, "out of control." He stated, "Fear of addiction makes one addicted. I kept taking it because I was so afraid not to take it." He was not able to wean completely off and instead remained on low dose Suboxone and continued doing well with his life in spite of ongoing, but lessened pain. He also stated that he had tremendous support and strength from his wife and from his God.

Zachary, a forty-nine year old man, had a low back fusion surgery at two levels two times. He was on opioids for a couple years but wanted to get off them "because I just don't feel like myself and I'm sick of how they make me feel. I get irritable easily. Also I'm sick of how I am treated in society, like I'm a drug seeker." It took a long time to wean down slowly from Oxycontin 30 mg every eight hours. On his first day off the opioids he stated, "Withdrawal makes you feel like pain is coming from deep within your bones... things that were suppressed are coming out...agitated, talkative, anxious...like a healing pain, not hard and sharp."

How much of the difficulties described above originate from external stimuli versus internal stimuli? Do external triggers prompt certain thoughts and feelings which in turn prompt further desires and behaviors? What underlying personal foundations, characteristics, temperaments, and personality traits and features are significantly influenced by various stimuli? What is actually pathological and not so easily changed? What is changeable?

Personality Disorders

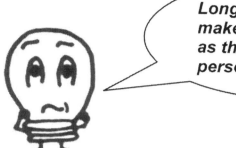

Long-term pain can make a person behave as though they have a personality disorder.

Just because you have chronic pain does not mean you are going crazy, although you may feel like it at times. Personality disorders are different from personality traits. We all have personality traits. These are defined by descriptive characteristics that in reality may include hypersensitivity to various stimuli, and in turn, hyperreactivity as well. Personality traits, in general, involve features that are pervasive across a wide range of life situations, activities, and social and personal contexts. Personality traits include enduring patterns of perceiving, thinking about, and relating to the environment and oneself. They are quite inflexible. They come on in late adolescence or early adulthood.

Personality traits become disorders when they markedly deviate from the expectations of a person's culture and are manifested in at least two of the domains of cognition (thinking), affectivity (feelings), interpersonal functioning (relationships), and/or impulse control. To be called a disorder they must also lead to clinically significant distress or impairment in social, occupational, or other important domains. They must not be caused by another mental disorder or be the direct physiological effect of chemicals or other medical problems.

The personality disorders are formally divided into three clusters. These include the formal Cluster A with descriptive characteristics such as odd and idiosyncratic thinking, suspiciousness, and social withdrawal. The formal Cluster B involves descriptive characteristics such as intense emotional experience and expression, poor impulse control, poor frustration tolerance, and mood swings. The formal Cluster C involves descriptive characteristics such as anxiety, worry, emotional constriction, poor decision-making, poor risk-taking, dependency, and excessive avoidance of pain and discomfort.

The person with a personality disorder may have fewer internal resources to deal with stress. This would make the person more sensitive and hyperresponsive to stress than a person without a personality disorder. This is called the ***stress diathesis model***. It means that the person has an underlying condition or weakness that makes it more difficult for them to handle an additional stress or difficulty.

The use of clinical descriptive characteristics as described in the three clusters A, B, C above are the formal way to think about and differentiate the various personality disorders. There are more specific descriptive characteristics for each of the specific personality disorders in each of the three clusters. However, in reality, personality disorders involve more than simple lists of descriptive characteristics. They are outward manifestations of internal biological processes that in actuality are unique to each unique individual human being. Brain parts and networks are involved. There are biological phenomena which we can only guess at. Our guesses, to a degree, and as described, are probably accurate. But they are probably incomplete.

There are three disorders described in cluster A and they all have certain descriptive characteristics in common. They are ***paranoid***, ***schizoid***, and ***schizotypal***. They all involve idiosyncratic thinking, suspiciousness, and social withdrawal. These features may be the result of limbic system and particularly amygdala hypersensitivity and hyper-responsiveness. The paranoid person may be hypersensitive to and misinterpret others' actions. The schizoid person may be uncomfortable or hypersensitive to being around other people. He or she may actually be fairly indifferent and insensitive to others. The schizotypal person may experience peculiarities of ideation, may demonstrate peculiar appearance, and may struggle with behaviors and deficits in interpersonal relationships. This person's pervasive pattern of social and interpersonal deficits may be marked by acute discomfort or hypersensitivity to, or reduced capacity for, close relationships.

There are four particular disorders in cluster B and they all have certain descriptive characteristics in common. They are *antisocial, borderline, histrionic*, and *narcissistic*. They all involve intense emotional experience and expression, mood swings, poor impulse control, and poor frustration tolerance. These features may be the result of limbic system and particularly amygdala hypersensitivity and hyper-responsiveness. These four disorders also seem to describe persons who lack sensitivity to the feelings and needs of others. They may be more sensitive and more focused on their own needs and lack of satisfaction in life.

Further descriptive characteristics of antisocial personality disorder include a pervasive pattern of disregard for, or violation of, the rights of others, a reckless disregard for the safety of self or others, and lack of remorse. This might imply a lack of sensitivity to others' feelings and needs. It might imply a hypersensitivity and hyperreactivity to one's own level of discomfort and need.

Borderline personality disorder involves instability in interpersonal relationships, instability in self-image, and affective instability. There are frantic efforts to avoid real or imagined abandonment. Marsha Linehan, psychologist at the University of Washington, and one of the world's leading experts on borderline personality disorder, describes: "Borderline individuals are the psychological equivalent of third-degree burn patients. They simply have, so to speak, no emotional skin. Even the slightest touch or movement can create intense suffering." This comment was also quoted by John Cloud in his article for Time Magazine, *Your Brain: A Users Guide*, 2009, as he described the suffering that borderline personality disordered people feel. They are definitely hypersensitive to the sense of rejection or possible separation from others. This is felt to be associated with the chronic feelings of emptiness.

The person with histrionic personality disorder struggles with a pattern of excessive emotionality and attention seeking. The person is uncomfortable in situations in which he or she is not the center of attention. Among other descriptive characteristics these persons may consider relationships to be more intimate than they actually are. This also might imply a lack of sensitivity to the feelings and experiences of others and more sensitivity and hyperreactivity to one's own discomfort and need.

The person with narcissistic personality disorder demonstrates a pervasive pattern of grandiosity, need for attention, and lack of empathy. This lack of empathy is further described in the DSM as "unwilling to recognize or identify with the feelings and needs of others." Based on biological considerations, one might wonder if the person is actually *unable* to recognize or identify with the feelings and needs of others. He or she also may experience a significant sense of entitlement, and be interpersonally exploitative, taking advantage of others to achieve his or her own ends. This again implies a lack of sensitivity to the needs and feelings of others, which in turn might imply a hypersensitivity to one's own sense of dissatisfaction in life, and a hypersensitivity to, and lack of awareness of, one's own sense of emptiness and need.

There are three particular disorders in cluster C and all have certain descriptive characteristics in common. These are ***avoidant***, ***dependent***, and ***obsessive-compulsive***. They all involve an underlying sense of perpetual or fairly consistent anxiety, worry about many things, emotional constriction or limitation or guardedness, poor decision making, unwillingness to take risks, dependency, and excessive avoidance of pain or change. Like the other personality disorders, these features may be the result of, or at least partly related to, limbic system and particularly amygdala hypersensitivity and hyper-responsiveness.

For example, a person with avoidant personality disorder will be hypersensitive to potential rejection, humiliation, or shame. A person with dependent personality disorder will be dependent and submissive, feeling very uncomfortable when asked to make decisions or even to be responsible for major areas of his or her own life. This person would be hypersensitive to the thought of being alone. The person with obsessive-compulsive personality disorder would be consistently perfectionistic and inflexible. In reality, this person would be hypersensitive to "imperfection" and unable to tolerate inefficiency, ambiguity, and uncertainty. This person would be unwilling to delegate, would be preoccupied with rules, lists, order, and organization to the extent that the major point of the activity would be lost.

All the personality disorders demonstrate some level of insensitivity (although probably lack of awareness) to other people and hypersensitivity to one's own feelings, desires, cravings, needs, dissatisfactions, and discomforts. Again, long-term pain can make a person behave as though they have a personality disorder.

PART 3:

PAIN PROBLEMS LIFE SOLUTIONS

GENERAL MEDICAL IDEAS AND APPROACHES

"Fresh thinking is hard to do. We are creatures of habit. You can come to realize, 'This is where I'm at, how can I build on my strengths?' This is what rehabilitation is all about. I have this chronic pain. Is there anything I can do to get the best quality of life?"
  MATTHEW MONSEIN, MD

"My wife is my saving grace."
  PATIENT

"You have to make a decision about how much you want to let the pain stop you from being who you want to be."
  PATIENT

"Sometimes the receptors in your brain tell your body there is no pain. Sometimes your body listens. Sometimes it doesn't listen. It barks back."
  PATIENT

The person in pain goes to the doctor with the hope and expectation that the medical problem can be found, and fixed. The person wants to be done with it and move on with life. However, many medical problems, and particularly neuropathic pain, are very complex, difficult to diagnose and understand, difficult to fix, and can really complicate the person's life, even long-term.

Nicole, a forty year old woman with long-term back and neck pain and a great deal of medical experience trying to lessen the pain, stated, "Pain feels like I am falling out of the sky and screaming for help before I hit the ground. I need help with the hysteria. I feel intensely desperate. I am not able to think clearly. My whole life is destroyed. All the opioids and other drugs, all the physical therapies and injections, and even surgeries are used out of a frantic, anxious, hopeful, wild search for relief."

Colleen, a thirty-seven year old woman who had been severely bitten by a dog on her right arm, stated that her muscles felt like they were "pulling on a steel cable." It was "extreme discomfort, not really pain," she stated. She said it felt like the muscles were "made of stone, exploding pressure." Neurontin seemed to work on these sensations. The sensation was "nasty and intense," she stated. She also stated that rehabilitation seemed to become easier "when there are no other choices."

There are basically four main things that the medical profession can do for the person dealing with pain. These include various surgeries, injections, many forms of physical therapies, and medications. These can work well for acute and subacute pain. For a person struggling with long-term pain, most of the medical treatment approaches tend to give temporary relief. There is nothing wrong with temporary relief. A person suffering with the pain might truly welcome some temporary relief. There may be a great deal of pain and suffering that can be calmed significantly, although usually temporarily, by various treatment approaches. A patient described taking her Percocet. She stated, "I can feel it coming on. Then it blocks out everything. This is good for the time being, but it is not a long-term plan for this long-term problem."

There is also a difference between passive and active treatment approaches. Passive treatment approaches require the patient to simply show up and receive the treatment. The treatment is actually done by someone else. The person dealing with long-term pain knows, generally, that the things that are done passively to the person tend to give temporary relief. This is not always true, of course. Sometimes passive therapies can give long-term benefit. Massage, heat, and ultrasound might help facilitate more success with the gentle ongoing active exercise plan. The hot tub before and after laps of swimming might help keep the muscles more loose and relaxed. Usually, however, when dealing with long-term problems, the passive therapies tend to give temporary relief at best. Sometimes the passive therapies don't work at all or even make things worse.

Treatment approaches that involve the active participation of the patient tend to give more long-term benefit. Active approaches usually need to be used in order to facilitate long-term benefit. When you have a long-term problem you will probably need treatment approaches that facilitate long-term benefits.

The four medical approaches listed, surgeries, injections, physical therapies, and medications, are what the medical profession can do for you. Active approaches are the many things that you might be able to do for yourself. Active approaches may include physical exercise. This will most likely involve slow, gentle, gradual, consistent exercises for specific body parts that hurt. This will also involve general body endurance building.

Active also means using relaxation or mental imagery approaches. These can look fairly passive, but indeed, the person is actually doing the activity instead of something simply being done to the person.

Active also means making small steps to solve problems. No one can do this for you. This has to be done by you. Active small steps are actually some of the best stress management techniques. Big steps might be something like, "If you are out of a job, get a job; if you have pain, get rid of pain." If these are not possible, then small steps may have to be utilized.

Learning is active. A student in the classroom who simply sits passively in the back of the room with his head back and says "teach me" probably will not learn as well as the student in front who pays attention, asks questions, and studies the material in an active manner. Active learning has more potential for the long-run.

The active approaches may involve the whole process of changing the mental and physical paradigm concerning how you view and experience the pain. The meaning and suffering components need to be recognized, contemplated, and possibly changed. New pathways in the brain and the brain/body need to be formed. The amygdala and anterior cingulate cortex need to be calmed and comforted. The frontal lobe and the hippocampus need to be strengthened and fortified. The sympathetic nervous system needs to be quieted and relaxed. The parasympathetic nervous system needs to be activated. The pain transmitting chemicals need to be blocked and the pain blocking chemicals need to be enhanced.

New activities need to be planned and practiced. New goals need to be made and accomplished. If you keep striving only to make pain less, but have no other goals, you may waste a lot of time and energy. You may need to keep striving for less pain. This is a good and appropriate goal. But there may need to be other goals as well.

Learning something new, seeing yourself doing, functioning, and accomplishing things, even with the pain onboard, might help create and strengthen new pathways in the nervous system and body. For example, when setting up for a golf swing, the golfer puts weight on one foot and then shifts to the other, and then back and forth, also adjusting his hands and arms and head over and over until it *feels* right. He does this until he *feels* the hit of the ball before he hits it. This is learned sensitivity with respect to hitting a golf ball. Might it be that a person has learned this sensitivity in dealing with long-term pain, and that the person then becomes too cautious in doing activities for fear of worsening or being flared up with pain? Can it be that new pathways of confidence with respect to doing various activities can be formed with practice?

It seems that there are a number of things that you can do to bring about significant change, to improve your life, to increase function, and possibly even to lessen pain. One thing might be to change the goal from "lessening pain" to "lessening suffering and increasing life." Physical exercise, including specific body part exercises and general body endurance building, can be helpful. Mental exercises including relaxation/imagery, biofeedback, meditation, breathing techniques, progressive muscle relaxation techniques, and mindfulness can all be helpful. Combinations of physical and mental techniques like yoga, tai chi, and qui gong can be very effective. There are many psychological therapies and approaches that can facilitate long-term benefits. The following illustrate various fascinating and remarkable techniques to change the hypersensitivity and hyperreactivity of the nervous system.

Other Ideas And Approaches

✓ *Systematic Desensitization*
✓ *Mirror Neuron System Theory/Therapy*
✓ *Salience Landscape Theory/Therapy*
✓ *Constraint Induced Movement Therapy*
✓ *Support and Structure*
✓ *Dialectical Behavior Therapy*
✓ *Spirituality*
✓ *Calming the Sympathetic Nervous System*

Before successful rehabilitation, the patients struggling with long-term pain have life goals that seem very focused, limited, and straight forward: to lessen pain. They can hardly focus on anything else. If they are asked about their mission in life or purpose in life, they state something about the pain and its effects on their life.

After successful rehabilitation, when they are asked about their mission or purpose in life, they usually don't even mention pain. The following quotes are examples:

"Since the pain program my mission is now to take care of my family and make sure they are safe and happy in life. I plan to get our house built. I was hurt on the job. I had three unsuccessful back surgeries. I was horizontal for two years. Finally I went through pain rehabilitation. I am now up and about and functioning. I have returned to part time work, and I am not depressed. I am hopeful."

Another patient whose life also seemed destroyed by her injury, pain, and her own responses stated that her goal was "to contribute in personal life as well as society as a whole, and to get back to some normalcy."

Another said he wanted "to help keep kids off the streets by raising money to keep them in other activities, to help them to have a better outlook on life." He also stated that he was "not going to follow old friends and habits by using hard drugs any longer."

Another stated, "I want to live everyday as full as I can, and be grateful for every little thing even if it is as little as a hug or a sip of water; just being able to tell my mom and dad that I love them more than anything."

A woman who lost her job, but believed she could find work again, did so, and stated, "I want to bring a smile to every face I meet. I want to tell people that this is it. You only get one chance at life. Don't waste it. Do only things that make you and those you love happy. Don't waste time feeling sorry for yourself."

How did these people do this? What kinds of things did they do to really change their paradigms? Were there dramatic epiphanies? What did they do with their own attitudes, adjustments, and behavior modifications to make such significant differences?

They all did many different things, and that's the point. In rehabilitation they re-scripted new lives. They practiced and learned new thoughts, new feelings, and new behaviors that eventually changed things for the better. Practicing new things brought about biological, biochemical changes in their brain/bodies. Amygdalae were calmed. Hippocampi were strengthened. Sympathetic activity was softened. Neurons were trained to sensitize to natural, endogenous antidepressant, antianxiety, and pleasurable chemicals. Normal sleep pathways were restored. Neurons were habituated somewhat to the painful inputs. The new thoughts, feelings, and behaviors were life-saving.

Systematic Desensitization

This involves a systematic approach to hopefully desensitize the person to a particular stimulus and to change the person's usual responses. Exposure with response prevention is the psychological jargon officially used. A person may be exposed to or encounter a particular stimulus such as seeing a mouse run across the kitchen floor. A response might be to jump up on the chair and scream. Systematic desensitization involves seeing the mouse and practicing sitting quietly in the chair. Exposure to a particular stimulus and prevention of a particular response is the general idea. A person who is afraid in elevators may really want to get off the elevator. A person who feels that germs are covering his hands may repetitively wash his hands. The person who experiences pain at work may want to leave work.

Exposure with response prevention can be practiced systematically, a little at a time. The person may have become abnormally sensitive to the particular stimulus or situation. Neurons, their receptors, and brain/body pathways may have become sensitized to pain and associated feelings, thoughts and behaviors. The person feels anxiety or pain, practices a particular escape activity or behavior, and then feels relief which reinforces the escape behavior. He becomes an expert at this brain/body habitual pattern. In order to change the person's life, the pattern may need to be changed. This may have to be done gradually.

In Pavlov's classical conditioning model a bell is rung just before meat is given to the dog. When presented with the meat the dog salivates naturally. But the dog also eventually learns and salivates when simply hearing the bell. The meat is the unconditioned stimulus. It didn't require any learning to bring about the response of salivation. The bell is the conditioned stimulus. It required learning, conditioning, to bring about the response of salivation.

This phenomenon does not just occur in dogs. A person can be presented with a conditioned stimulus just before an unconditioned stimulus as well. In the pain situation, a person might experience the thought of the job where he was hurt and develop the response of muscle tightness in the body. Even the site or thought of the workplace where injury occurred, certain smells, sounds, relationships, and many other stimuli in this workplace can bring on worsened pain. This is learned. The brain/body neurobiochemical pathways are stimulated, set in motion, and result in further painful experiences. The person behaves in certain natural ways when hurting and can learn to behave in these ways when exposed to the environment where the pain was originally experienced or worsened. The person can be taught to have the same brain/body responses when exposed to the conditioned stimulus only.

Conditioned Stimulus	Unconditioned Stimulus	Biological Response	Behavioral Response	Reinforcer of the Response
Bell	Meat	Saliva	Eat	Feel good
Something in the environ. (internal or external)	Thought of germs on hands	Anxiety	Wash hands	Feel relief
Something in the environ. (internal or External)	Thought of work	Pain, Anxiety, Depression, Anger, Muscle tightness, Neurobiological Physiological Responses	Behaviors to avoid worse pain, drug use, going to bed	Feel relief

Systematic desensitization is a technique used to extinguish or lessen responses associated with exposure to a particular situation. Systematic desensitization is used in many rehabilitation and pain management approaches. A person is advised to exercise slowly and gently, trying to find a middle ground or moderate level of activity somewhere between doing too much and doing too little. The person is advised to practice the exercise and prevent the normal response of quitting. Eventually this may help lessen and/or extinguish certain pain behaviors.

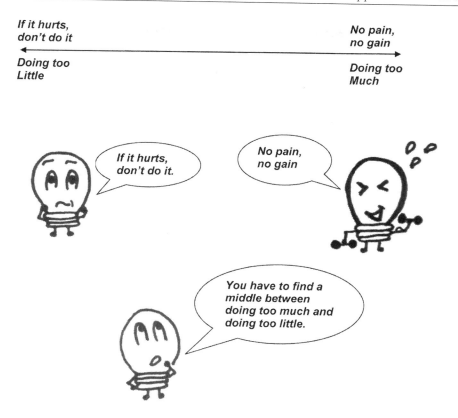

"No pain, no gain" will not work well for many people struggling with long-term pain. A neurologist, making a referral to a pain program, wrote in the referral letter, "I want this person in a vigorous, strenuous exercise program." The physician had the idea that somehow ignoring the pain, blasting through the pain, would be significantly beneficial. Our culture, in general, and the neurologist specifically, is hard-driving, strong-willed, and determined. One might also hear or sense the underlying intent of punishment, of blaming the victim, in this statement from the neurologist. This could come from the neurologist feeling frustrated about not being able to make the person better with standard medical approaches. Possibly the neurologist also believed that the patient was not trying or was being coddled by therapists in the past. Or the neurologist really believed that strenuous exercise would work. Maybe he was right. Maybe not.

"If it hurts, don't do it" is the opposite approach and won't work well for chronic pain problems either. The person may hurt when doing nothing, like lying in bed, eating a meal, or doing very simple activities. Indeed, the person is not causing any further tissue damage. Again, exposure to the exercise and functional activities and the prevention of the normal avoidance responses, may help to lessen and/or extinguish certain pain behaviors.

We might ask in the group setting at the pain clinic, "Do you hurt now?" The patients, of course, all say "yes" even though they are simply sitting there in the group and doing nothing that would worsen the underlying physical pathology or cause further physical harm. The facilitator might joke, "Then stop doing that." The patients routinely understand the issue here. Again, they are not doing anything wrong in that moment to cause tissue damage. In this situation, "if it hurts, don't do it" does not apply.

A person may be advised to return to work on a graduated basis. Exposure to the workplace slowly, gradually, and with the prevention of leaving or escape may lead to extinction of the neurobiological, physiological experiences such as anxiety and its physical symptoms and signs. It may lead to the extinction of the neurobiological, physiological problems of depression, anger, and muscle tightness. Pain might actually lessen over time and practice, as long as the person is not doing things on the job that are actually causing tissue damage or are unsafe due to the underlying medical problem. With practice the person can find the middle ground between doing too much and doing too little.

Another psychologically minded patient wondered if the physical pain he was experiencing at work was somehow symbolic of his perceived sense of injustice in the situation. His supervisor and fellow employees were critical of him since his injury and return to work. They did not trust him and he did not trust them. He was also given only meaningless non-productive work with no prospect of improvement in the situation, as far as he could tell. He was bored, angry, and depressed. But he was also insightful as he asked the question about his pain and its worsening at work.

We are all aware of the fact that positive reinforcers are things that make it more likely that a particular behavior will occur again. One's paycheck at the end of the week keeps the person coming back to work the next week. M&Ms or praise might encourage the child to do a particular activity again. The child is rewarded for asking politely for things. The child is rewarded for saying thank you. The child is rewarded systematically during toilet training.

The strongest positive reinforcement schedules include random, intermittent use of the positive reinforcers. If the person is reinforced consistently, always the same all the time, the likelihood of performing that activity again is increased but it is increased even more if the person is reinforced more randomly or intermittently. This is the typical reinforcement schedule in golf, for most golfers, when only occasionally, randomly, and intermittently does the person have a really good shot. This is also true in gambling, fishing, and many other almost addicting activities. This is the most powerful and addictive behavior reinforcement schedule. In addiction behavior certain pathways in the brain, spinal cord, and brain/body connections becomes deeply etched, imprinted, and carved like a "groove" or a "rut." The person becomes stuck in a certain pattern of behavior. "If you always do what you always did, you'll always get what you always got."

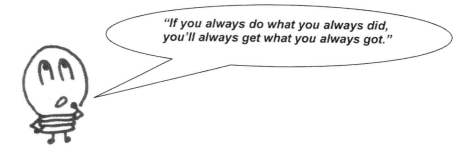

"If you always do what you always did, you'll always get what you always got."

In the painful experience, the feeling of relief, slightly less pain, slightly less anxiety and increased sense of calm, slightly less muscle tightness, all become the positive reinforcers for the pain behaviors. The pain behaviors of drug use and inactivity are reinforced by feeling better. Wouldn't it be nice to experience this similar sense of relief, slightly less pain, slightly less anxiety, slightly less muscle tightness, more muscle relaxation and increased sense of calm when using other techniques mentally and physically?

The person may have to practice different techniques. The person may have to practice exposure to activities that seem to increase pain somewhat. The person may have to prevent the natural avoidant responses. This does not mean that the person should cause tissue damage to the body by doing too much. "No pain, no gain" does not apply. On the other hand, it doesn't mean that the person should not do things that hurt at all. "If it hurts, don't do it" does not apply fully either. It simply means that the person needs to change the previous pattern of activity. The person needs to avoid avoiding.

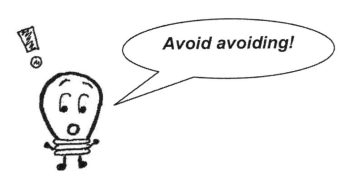

In summary, systematic desensitization is a technique used to extinguish or lessen responses associated with exposure to a particular situation. The responses may be normal and natural but not necessarily helpful. Therefore, it might be best to change those natural responses. The patient in pain responds with pain behaviors, like taking drugs and going to bed when flared-up. This does not usually work well in the long run for long-term pain problems. In fact, these behaviors gradually tend to make things worse. Therefore, changes need to be made. Changing what you can in terms of thoughts, feelings, and behaviors will result in neurobiological, biochemical changes that can make a difference in the long run.

Mirror Neuron Theory/Therapy

For decades we've known that certain "primary motor neurons" in the primary motor cortex or motor strip fire when an animal is executing or carrying out an activity or physical movement. The primary motor neurons in the brain are where the activity actually begins. The messages are then sent down from these neurons through the brain and nervous system to the muscles to make the activity happen. This is true when a monkey reaches for a peanut. This is true when a person sings a song, wiggles a finger, drinks a cup of coffee, and pushes to have a bowel movement. This is true when you are doing anything and everything.

In the 1990's, researchers discovered that there are some other very special neurons (not just the primary motor neurons) that fire when the monkey reaches for the peanut. Also, these same special neurons fire when the monkey is simply watching another person or monkey performing the same function. It is like the little neuron cannot tell the difference between seeing and doing.

This neuron and others like it are located in many parts of the brain. Two of the parts are the ***premotor cortex*** and the ***supplementary motor areas*** of the brain's frontal lobe.

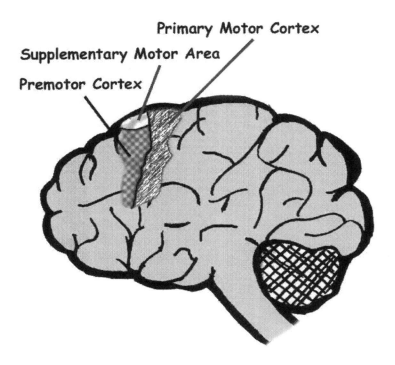

Primary Motor Cortex

Supplementary Motor Area

Premotor Cortex

The neurons in the primary motor cortex or motor strip fire when the person or primate reaches for the peanut, as do the neurons in front of the primary motor strip, the premotor cortex and supplementary motor cortex. The neurons in the premotor cortex and supplementary motor cortex also fire when the primate simply sees another animal reach for the peanut. These neurons fire when a person even *thinks* about the action. These neurons are called "mirror neurons."

Two other areas of interest where mirror neurons are located are the anterior cingulate cortex and the ***insular cortex***. The anterior cingulate cortex is active in a wide variety of cognitive and emotional tasks, and the insular cortex is involved in a great deal of subjective emotional experience. The insular cortex is also involved in processing information about attention, music, eating and all of our five senses.

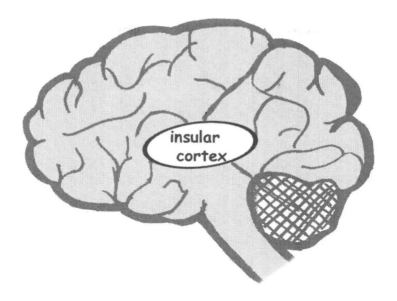

In humans these mirror neurons also seem to be related to empathy, cognitions, and feelings, not just motor movements. They help us feel, sense, and experience what others feel. The mirror neurons help us to feel what another person is feeling without actually going through the same specific experience. For example, mirror neurons in and around the anterior cingulate cortex fire when a person is in pain. For most of us, the same neurons fire when a person sees someone else in pain. A patient said one time, "It hurts me to watch someone else get a shot." Of course, most of us do not actually feel the exact same pain that another person feels. But we might feel the anxiety, fear, frustration, anger, and sadness more clearly. Some might actually feel physical pain.

One hypothesis concerning persons lacking empathy is that they may not have fully developed or fully active mirror neuron systems or networks. The mirror neurons normally have functions which involve monitoring and being sensitive to various actions and movements of one's own self and of others. These neurons work in tandem with other parts of one's nervous system. As stated earlier, when various parts of the nervous system are functioning together, they are called networks. At times there may be something wrong with the networks. If cheese is made in a particular town and another town does not receive its weekly shipment of cheese, one might conclude that there is something wrong in the cheese factory itself. However, maybe there is nothing wrong with the factory. Maybe the problem is that there is something wrong with the road from the factory or from one town to the other. Or maybe there is something wrong with the trucks that deliver the cheese, or the road signs, or the weather, or many other possible problems. The nervous system networks are like this. What is actually and specifically going on when a person is hurting and suffering is usually unclear.

When we watch American Idol, Dancing with the Stars, or Monday Night Football the person watching is in reality, in their own brain and nervous system, feeling what the participants are feeling. The person is essentially almost there, almost the one actually doing the activity.

Mirror neuron networks and systems help us think about something, feel something, and then as a result, send messages to motor neurons to do something. I see the spider, feel fear, and then move away. There is another psychological theory, the *James-Lange theory*, that describes this process occurring in a different order. It states that one might see the spider, move away from the spider, and then feel the fear. However, in the pain situation, or a work injury situation for example, one might imagine that the person who has been injured on the job might later see the job, feel fear and pain, and then try to move away from the job situation.

The mirror neuron networks and systems help us to be sensitive to another person's movements, thoughts, and feelings. They are involved in empathy, understanding, and feeling what someone else feels. But not only are the mirror neurons involved in the sense of "compassion" or "suffering with" another, it seems that they also help us to be aware or sensitive to the intentions of another person. They help us to anticipate what someone else might do at a particular time or in a particular situation.

In primates the mirror neuron systems seem to be only helpful in predicting simple goal directed behaviors. We do not know this for sure, but this is what can be measured or scientifically studied and monitored so far. In humans the mirror neuron systems may be helpful in predicting and understanding more complex behaviors and intentions.

The ***angular gyrus*** is another brain part where mirror neurons have been found.

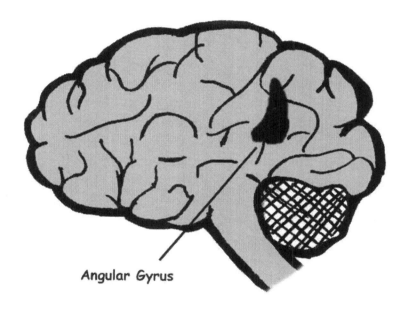

Angular Gyrus

This brain part is an associative area or an area that sits at the intersection or junction of the brain's vision, hearing, and touch centers. It helps bind together the various senses. We can experience an apple fully because when we bite into it, we can enjoy its sweet-tart *taste*, crisp-cold texture and *touch*, bright-red *color*, tangy-citrus *smell*, and the crackling *sound* all at once. As we bite and chew, all of our senses are stimulated at once. The chewing movements can be pleasurable as they continue to be paired with the other pleasurable sensations. We can practice and become very sensitive to this fully pleasurable experience of all the senses and motor activities at once. We can also think ahead and experience the knowledge of the health that the apple will bring for the future. The present and the future can be paired together and can be pleasurable together. With practice we can etch these brain patterns and networks deeply into the brain. We can become sensitive to this experience. It might not take much stimulus to actually feel the pleasure. We might be able to feel the pleasure simply by thinking about the apple-eating experience or watching someone else eat the apple.

When we feed a baby, we open our mouths as if we were almost taking in the food ourselves. As the baby watches you open your mouth, he might then open his mouth as well. It seems that mirror neuron systems are very active when feeding another person.

The November 2006 issue of Scientific American described a mirror neuron theory of **autism**. It raised very interesting questions about the possible biological underpinnings of autism. It talked about the fact that many children with autism may have normal intelligence but profound deficits in social interactions. Certain brain functions and activities can be studied by doing EEG monitoring while the person does a simple activity such as opening and closing the hand. This can be compared to brain activity when the person simply watches someone else perform the same physical actions. For most people, the brain wave patterns for doing and seeing look about the same. For someone with autism, the brain wave patterns do not look the same. It is thought that there may be something wrong with the mirror neuron systems.

For most of us, connections with other people feel good. Patients with chronic pain typically become less social, do less and less with friends, coworkers, and family, and tend to isolate themselves. This does not help anything. It can make things worse. In order to feel better in life the person in pain needs to connect with other people who feel the same or similar things. Again, finding a middle ground between doing too much with other people and not doing anything with anybody is very important.

Is seeing "eye to eye" possibly associated with stimulating the mirror neuron systems in both people? Does simply making eye contact stimulate the mirror neuron systems in both people? Are we able to understand something about another's intensions and feelings and thoughts by making eye contact? Can a person feel better by helping someone else, by doing something good for someone else? Can a person feel better by simply connecting with someone else, feeling the empathy and caring of someone else, even a pet? Can one feel better by experiencing someone else's pain with a sense of compassion, caring, and sensitivity?

People are often "caretaking." This means that they tend to take care of other people even to the detriment of taking care of themselves. When you do something nice for someone else, it can feel good to you. Can volunteerism be a way to stimulate your mirror neuron system, increase your own pleasure and enjoyment in life, and possibly even lessen pain and suffering?

As stated, the mirror neurons are parts of networks and systems. They can be parts of pain sensitivity systems and networks, but also parts of pleasure sensitivity systems and networks. You can practice using the systems and networks that are helpful to you as opposed to only those that are not so helpful in the long run.

Do the things that you can do for someone else, things that you actually can do without hurting yourself. One thing you can do, though it may be very difficult as we tend to be very independent, self-sufficient people, is to let someone else care for you. Letting someone else care for you can be a gift to that other person, just as it would be a gift to you, to let you care for someone else. Be sure to thank them.

Salience Landscape Theory/Therapy

What you *think* about and *feel* most of the time, *with whom you associate* most of the time, and *what activities you participate in* most of the time become the background and foundation of all your experiences. They become the landscape on the canvas of the picture of your life. You are in the foreground but your surrounding family members, friends, recreational activities, where you live, what you eat and drink, your vacations, dreams, memories and experiences are all parts of your salient landscape. Even your *self-talk*, what you say to yourself most of the time, about yourself, is part of this landscape.

Ideas about one's salient landscape were described in the November 2006 Scientific American article discussing theories of autism. These ideas were developed in collaboration with William Hirsten of Elmhurst College and Portia Iversen of Cure Autism Now. It is interesting that studies on autism can give us insight into what might be happening in chronic pain. Ideas about one's salient landscape apparently might explain some of the repetitive behaviors and hypersensitivity of the person with autism and the hypersensitivity and repetitive behaviors of the person struggling with long-term pain.

During each waking moment of our lives, all of us are bombarded with many millions/billions of inputs through all our various senses, all at the same time. It has been said that at any given moment we are presented with 400 billion inputs of information at once. However, we can only attend to about two thousand at a time. This concept was presented in the movie, *What the Bleep Do We Know*, a *Captured Light Industries, Lord of the Wind* film that was first presented in 2004. This information, both the conscious and the subconscious, is transmitted deep into the brain and limbic system. These structures determine how we should react emotionally to the various inputs. In turn, these structures send information and messages to the autonomic nervous system which then feeds further information to other brain/body networks. Information is also sent to the thinking and planning networks and the motor activity networks. It is then sent back to the sensory networks and continues this repetitive, circular cycle of feedback information. Normally, if we do not have any specific attention deficit or other attentional difficulties, we attend to incoming information that is really important in the moment.

The autistic person may not be able to filter out or censor the less-than-important inputs in the moment. The nervous system will become overwhelmed by the massive amount of information at any one time. The person with autism is not able to focus and attend to only that information which is really important at any one time. The sensory information is relayed to the limbic system and then to the autonomic nervous system and to other brain and nervous system networks. The emotional content is noted and emotion regulation is activated. The person with autism may be hypersensitive to the massive amount of sensory information at any one time. The person may not be able to block out the majority of the sensory input. The person may not be able to attend to a limited number of inputs at once.

Imagine you are in a noisy restaurant and are trying to listen to the person in the booth with you. Imagine that you are not able to block out the other patrons and noises. It could become overwhelming and you might want to cover your ears totally. Thus persons with some types of autism may avoid eye contact, not want to be hugged, desire more solitude, and not really connect with other people. It is just too much coming in at once and can't be filtered.

Normally, we are able to develop a background of experience, emotion, thought, and expression that is consistent with all the knowledge and inputs that have been stored, consolidated, and coordinated all through our lives. Normally, we are able to decide what is important and deal with what is important in any particular moment and in any particular situation. Normally, there are active connections between the sensory inputs to the limbic system, and active connections from the limbic system to the frontal cortex for foresight and planning. Normally, there are active connections between the limbic system and the sympathetic nervous system, from the amygdala to the motor strips for movement and responding; and between the sensory strips and mirror neuron systems for further consideration and experience. Over a lifetime of experience the limbic system constantly creates and stores a salience landscape. This becomes an ever-changing dictionary that details the emotional definitions, meanings, and significance of everything in the individual's experience.

However, if there are somehow disruptions or abnormal changes in the patterns of brain and nervous system activity, the person may experience sensory inputs abnormally and thus respond abnormally. The person may develop abnormal connections between the various brain networks. The person may respond to even trivial stimuli with extreme emotion and avoidance behaviors.

How does a person's salience landscape become so distorted? What happens to the brain and the rest of the nervous system when repetitious inputs of pain are being continually paired with experiences that normally would not hurt? What happens to the brain and the rest of the nervous system when there is constant or at least repetitive pairing of autonomic and sympathetic inputs with the painful stimulus? What happens to the brain and the rest of the nervous system when even the thoughts of the painful stimulus, experience, and situation are paired with other thoughts, emotions, and behaviors?

Each person's nervous system is constantly changing. The nervous system of the person struggling with long-term pain changes for better or for worse every moment of every day. It can be very helpful for a person to mindfully attend to experiences and behaviors that ameliorate pain rather than obliviously, mindlessly, and inattentively participate in thoughts, feelings, and behaviors that tend to make pain worse.

Self-stimulation can be calming for many people. The sympathetic nervous system responses can be lessened when a person rocks back and forth, repetitively taps their hands, says words or phrases over and over, or even uses head or body repetitive activities. An infant calms down with rocking and singing and patting. As adults we often seem to calm down with repetitive activities like singing, drumming, running, walking, swimming, biking, channel surfing with the remote control, reading, focusing on breathing, smoking, chewing, eating, drinking, and many other activities. Many hobbies are calming.

Is the person with schizophrenia, as he talks to himself out loud, actually calming himself? Could hearing a song go around and around in your brain over and over all day be somehow calming for a person? Could these types of experiences be similar to each other?

The sensory inputs of the person dealing with long-term pain may become distorted with the emotional suffering and the overwhelming inputs of emotional and irrational colors, meanings, and landscapes in the background of the entire painful experience. There may be strong and abnormal connections between various brain parts and networks that define the meaning of the pain in pathological ways. The person experiences more than pain. The person experiences suffering. This is due to the connections that form between the sensory organs, the fibers transmitting the painful messages up the limbs, the spinal cord, the thalamus, the amygdala, the frontal lobe, the anterior cingulate cortex, the hippocampus, and all the other brain parts and networks described and not yet described in neuroscience. Can these connections and sensory distortions, the connections between physical and emotional sensitivity and responses, be changed with practice?

For the person dealing with long-term pain, the pain becomes the salient center or background landscape. The person changes associations with family members, lessens associations with friends and coworkers, does less for fun, eats, drinks, and sleeps differently, spends more time secluded, and thinks negative thoughts about oneself. The whole experience of pain involves more than just the pain but also the salient landscape of the meaning of pain as well. As pain becomes long-term suffering becomes significant.

A person's normal salient landscape is built through a lifetime of experience. Pain has its normal protective meanings and purposes. As the person experiences pain long-term the landscape is often modified to represent more and more suffering. The person becomes anxious about being anxious, about being depressed, about having pain, and about being out of control. What the person thinks about and feels most of the time, with whom the person associates most of the time, and what activities the person participates in most of the time become the landscape on the canvas. How you relate to family and friends, what you do for recreational activities, what you eat and drink, what you dream, remember and plan, and even your self-talk become the new landscape. This is the landscape that needs to be modified, improved, softened, painted, and viewed differently during a rehabilitation process. All these things can be changed to a degree. The person has control of all these things to a degree. All these things can make a difference in the painful experience. The "landscape" can be changed. The neurobiochemical underpinnings can be changed. Remember "neurons that fire together wire together?" Changes can be made.

Marie, a sixty year old woman, had several years of left shoulder pain and two shoulder surgeries that left her with pain and minimal motion in the shoulder. She was left handed and was having a terrible time grieving or mourning the loss of her left arm function. She was on opioids for several years and was in the process of weaning down and off. She described the idea that normally things in life can be irritating and frustrating at times. Then she stated that it seemed abnormal that simple little things would "get under my skin" and become overwhelming. She stated that "under all this, the high dose of medications gives me an emotional lift to help me tolerate the fact that surgery was unsuccessful." She stated that her "senses seem dulled by the medication." She stated, "The use of the medications seems to bring me up to some kind of baseline. They certainly don't make me high. Without them I am really down. With them I am sort of normal, but certainly not happy." During the process of weaning off the opioids, her senses became less dulled and grieving was more intense. She stated that all in all the pain was not more intense. She stated that it was difficult, but it felt better to go through a grieving process and eventually "let go" of what she couldn't really change. She described that it was "easier to let go when I was taking a hold of something else." She was focusing on her family, what she was able do, and what she was grateful for in her life.

After the pain program, even many years later, patients are sometimes asked, "What was the most important part of the program? What really helped you the most in your rehabilitation? What was the most helpful in getting you back to life?" They will usually answer, "The other patients, the friendships, the connection with other people who understand without having to explain everything, the connection with other people who know and believe and experience the same issues and feelings." This is the mirror neuron system, the salient landscape, the calming of the amygdala and the anterior cingulate cortex, the stimulation of pleasure networks, the production and flow of various neurotransmitters that help us to feel good or better in spite of pain.

Constraint Induced Movement Therapy

When pain comes onboard, the person automatically demonstrates or starts practicing pain behaviors. The person limps with a knee or hip problem, leans over or sideways with a back problem, protects and does not use an injured arm, and takes medication and goes to bed when bombarded by a headache. These and many other pain behaviors are natural, can occur without specific learning, and are essentially unconditioned.

However, to a degree, behaviors can also be conditioned, practiced, and learned. A person can *learn* to practice pain behaviors, *learn* to avoid certain activities, *learn* to avoid the use of the injured body part, and *learn* how to respond emotionally as well as physically to the pain and injury. The person then suffers from "*learned non-use*" as described by Norman Doidge, MD, in his book titled, *The Brain That Changes Itself.* He describes the work of Edward

Taub, PhD, on Constraint Induced Movement Therapy (CIMT) for persons dealing with stroke. This refers to the neuroplasticity of the brain and nervous system when learning and undergoing rehabilitation.

Taub works with patients six to ten hours per day for several weeks, and the patients continue to practice on their own long-term. Because the brain/body is a use-it-or-lose-it organ/system, one might expect that a person who has not used his or her brain/body normally for a long time might not be able to use it again in a normal way. A person with a left hemisphere stroke might not be able to use the right arm. The less the person uses the arm, the more he practices not using the arm, the harder it becomes to use the arm. However, Taub helps many patients routinely improve dramatically with rehabilitation even if their problem began a long time ago. Taub knows, as all of us know, that sometimes the stroke is so severe that the use of the arm or leg or speech is not going to return. But there are many cases where return of function is not out of the question.

Taub states, when describing certain cases, "The person could use the arm if he really tried. But he doesn't try because he has learned not to try. It is a conditioned response. The patient can go on week after week, month after month, not using the particular body part. It can become more and more powerful, overwhelmingly powerful, to not use the body part." He goes on to state that "one has to counter-condition this extremely strong tendency not to use the arm. Small, clumsy movements have to be endlessly repeated. Simply overcoming this non-use of the limb is not enough. One has to repeat the movement over and over and over again."

When a person is struggling with long-term pain, he or she may spend more and more time in bed. The longer the person spends in bed, the harder it is to get out of bed. The harder it is to get out of bed, the longer the person spends in bed.

In the pain management rehabilitation setting, the person is encouraged to use the brain/body in more and more normal ways in spite of the ongoing and long-term pain. The person learns to use the brain/body again. It may be in different ways than "normal" or before the onset of pain, but it can be improved compared to what it has become after the onset of pain.

The person is persuaded to practice using the injured body parts in incremental small steps. This type of training is called ***shaping***. The person is introduced to exercises, in spite of the pain problem, in a slow, gentle, gradual manner. The person needs to find the middle ground between doing too much and doing too little. The brain/body rewires with plastic changes in the nervous system that mark improvements in function. The patient is not allowed to do what he or she would like to do, such as go to bed and take a pill. Instead, the person attends classes, uses various exercises, and practices mental imagery and relaxation approaches. The person gradually is able to do more and more in spite of the pain and its effects on the person's life. The "plastic," changeable brain/body is rewired for healthy behaviors, thoughts and attitudes, feelings and emotional responses, instead of persisting in the unhealthy reality of pain, anger, frustration, anxiety, blame, worry, depression, deconditioning, chemical use and abuse, and non-functioning behaviors.

If one goes to a particular meeting at work or church each week and always sits in the same chair or pew, this becomes a pathway or pattern of brain/body activity and nervous system involvement which *feels* a certain way: comfortable and confident without much extra thought. Changing the sitting arrangement can *feel* wrong and new and possibly even difficult to deal with.

Try something new or different. Try a simple experiment, such as sitting in a room, meeting, in a different place than you are normally used to. One thing that you might notice is that anticipating the change may be a bigger deal than the actual change. You might not feel much different sitting in a different place, nor will the people around you. Wonder ahead of time what it might feel like to make the change. It may not be as difficult as you might think. This may seem like a small thing and an unrealistic approach when dealing with the significant and severe pain situation. Can you make the steps toward improvement in the pain management situation small as well?

The best stress management techniques involve small steps to solve problems. We can use diversion, exercise, relaxation and mental imagery techniques, or maybe take a vacation or give one's self a break from the situation. This is difficult in the pain situation which never really lets up. However, medication use, drugs, or alcohol are often ways in which the person may be able to escape or separate one's self from the situation. The separation is very temporary of course. More constructive small steps can lead to more long-term benefits. Small steps to solve problems can result in more long lasting benefits and no adverse side effects.

Structure And Support

When people leave the pain management program, we routinely advise that they have in place daily activities in a structured manner. What is on their schedule for Monday next week, and each day after that? People were involved in structure every day before the pain came onboard. People with long-term pain typically lose the structure in their lives after the pain comes onboard. Very structured activities in the pain management program are part of the rehabilitation process. The patients need to continue daily structure after the pain program or they will regress to the dysfunctional lifestyle that was present before the pain program. Rehabilitation needs to continue on a daily basis.

Support of other people is one of the most important aspects of rehabilitation. Before pain comes onboard most people have friends and family and coworkers. Most people have support in life. After the pain comes onboard most of these relationships change as the person is not able to participate normally in life activities.

Support is experienced once again in the pain management program. Usually each person feels the supportive, understanding connection with the other people in the program. They also feel the support of caring staff. This is healing. This needs to be continued after the program.

Dialectical Behavior Therapy

This is a form of cognitive behavioral therapy developed by Dr. Marsha Linehan in the 1970's and 1980's at the University of Washington. It implies using cognition and behaviors to change emotions, and ultimately to change how the person feels and functions in life and relationships. This system of therapy was devised to help persons dealing with Borderline Personality Disorder to control their emotion dysregulation and learn to function more normally in society and life. The therapy approaches can be very useful for other conditions, particularly where there is emotion dysregulation, a sense of invalidation, and a need to establish compromise and synthesis between opposing ideas and issues.

In the pain management situation, the person dealing with long-term pain is often struggling with emotion dysregulation. The person, in addition to pain, is often experiencing anger, depression, fear, anxiety, confusion, uncertainty, blame, guilt, and a sense of injustice, all associated with lack of control.

Also, since our society is very intolerant of long-term difficulties, there is often a sense of invalidation. Our society often expects and believes that medical technology should be able to find and fix the medical problems, and that if this has not been accomplished, the person in pain is the one who is at fault somehow. We tend to think that the problems the person is experiencing are not for real, fraudulent, malingering, factitious, or simply drug-seeking. We tend to think that the person is somehow psychologically impaired. Valid means real. Believing that the person/problem is not for real is invalidation.

Also, in the pain management situation, statements such as "If it hurts, don't do it" *and* "No pain, no gain" do not go together very well. Another example might be "we accept you just the way you are" *and* "you need to change." Finding a middle ground between these various dichotomies is part of dialectical behavior therapy. This is finding the compromise and synthesis of opposing ideas and issues. The use of the word *and* is part of this process and indicates that both ideas, both ways of thinking and functioning, can be true at the same time.

Dialectical thinking refers to viewing and thinking about issues and situations from multiple perspectives. In the pain situations the person dealing with pain is not the only one involved. The person in pain is the one who is *afflicted* with the condition. But there are also the persons who are *affected*, such as family members, friends, employers, fellow employees, insurance people, attorneys, vocational case managers, and medical care providers. The *afflicted* and the *affected* all have different views, perspectives, and goals. Sometimes they have opposing ideas and issues which need compromise and synthesis.

In dialectical behavior therapy there is a concept called "wise mind." This is the combination of the "the reason mind" and "the emotion mind."

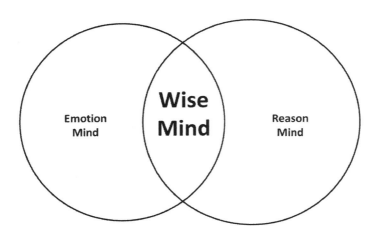

Sometimes the emotion mind can become extremely active and the reason mind can seem to be quite inactive.

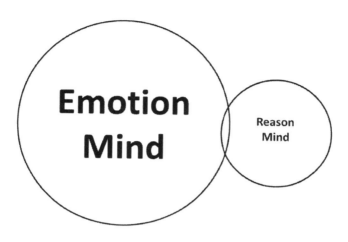

Sometimes the reason mind can seem extremely active and the emotion mind can seem quite inactive.

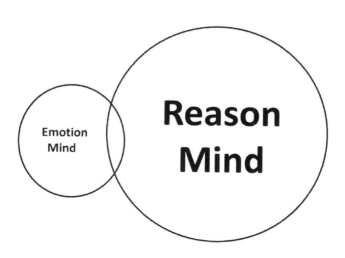

If one were to think of the particular brain parts that might be involved in these processes it might be as follows.

Emotion Mind

      Limbic system emotional networks

      Amygdala

      Anterior Cingulate Cortex

      Insular cortex

      (The three year old child who has a temper tantrum for almost no reason.)

Reason Mind

      Frontal Lobe

      Hippocampus

      (Logical, rigid, constant intellectualization, rationalization. A patient described the sense of "flat-lined:" no emotions, no sense of humor, no joy. This would be an extreme of course.)

Wise Mind

      Combination, balanced

      Part of the "wise mind" might include the list of "Assumptions About Borderline Patients and Therapy" as described by Dr. Marsha Linehan. Dr. Linehan's actual words might also apply when dealing with persons with Chronic Pain Syndrome.
1. "Patients are doing the best they can."
2. "Patients want to improve."
3. "Patients need to do better, try harder, and be more motivated to change."
4. "Patients may not have caused all of their own problems, but they have to solve them anyway."
5. "The lives of extremely depressed or anxious, suicidal individuals are unbearable as they are currently being lived."
6. "Patients must learn new behaviors in all relevant contexts."
7. "Patients cannot fail in therapy."
8. "Therapists treating patients need support."

EMDR and EFT and HYPNOSIS

EMDR is Eye Movement Desensitization and Reprocessing. EFT is Emotional Freedom Technique. Hypnosis is an induced altered state of consciousness, characterized by heightened suggestibility and receptivity. These three approaches involve techniques to ultimately change the feelings, thoughts, and behaviors of the person suffering with various physical and psychological difficulties. All involve the combinations of dialogue, focused attention, and re-patterning techniques. They all help a person to change patterns of feeling, thinking, and behaving that might be harmful or get in the way of a person's efforts to reach certain goals. If a person wants to lessen pain, but the person's emotions aggravate the pain, then the person might want to change the emotions. If a person's behaviors and thoughts aggravate the pain, then the person might want to change the behaviors and thoughts.

EMDR uses repetitive back and forth eye movements in association with concentration on the self-defeating thoughts or uncomfortable feelings in order to bring about change. It is used for reducing feelings of fear and anxiety as well as for strengthening feelings of calm and confidence. Desensitization is a process of becoming more comfortable with a memory or a feeling that is by itself uncomfortable. Reprocessing is a psychological term that means working on a thought, feeling, or memory to make it more useful and comfortable instead of just frightening or uncomfortable.

Emotional Freedom Techniques involve changing the emotions the person is experiencing so that the person is not so trapped by his or her experience and emotions. The techniques are based on several assumptions. Biological behavior can be controlled by invisible forces including thought. Every thought or emotion has a corresponding physical response. Our emotions and thoughts have a direct effect on our physical well-being, as well as our spiritual and mental well-being. The technique involves tapping parts of the body (acupoints) and thus changing brain activity. It is hoped that the procedure will deactivate areas of the brain that are involved with fear, anxiety, depression, and addictions. It is hoped that the procedure will activate other parts of the brain that have to do with health and comfort. Repetitive stimulation of body parts through tapping while bringing the trigger image or feeling to mind will be different than just experiencing the trigger image or feeling. It is felt that this difference can be helpful and beneficial.

Repetitive physical activities such as walking, jogging, drumming, or the rocking of a baby in the mother's arms all may be similar in their effects. They are often calming, relaxing, and change not only the body but also the brain. They can change the thoughts and feelings that the person is experiencing. A book by David Feinstein, Donna Eden, and Gary Craig, titled *The Promise of Energy Psychology: Revolutionary Tools for Dramatic Personal Change* describes EFT fully.

Hypnosis changes brain activity in many ways. The frontal lobes for foresight and planning, the anterior cingulate cortex for evaluating emotional components of an experience, and many sensory areas for blocking out pain at least temporarily can all be involved. Many other brain/body parts and networks can be involved. The brain doesn't just sit there receiving information from the body, painful or otherwise. The brain is involved in interpreting, responding to, changing, and sometimes even initiating various experiences. The brain is actually in charge of everything. How we think, the emotions we feel clearly or on a deep subconscious level, and the behaviors we practice all make a difference. Everything can be influenced by hypnosis.

Spirituality

Janine, a forty year old widowed woman with **Ehler's Danlos** and severe pain in her joints and muscles, said, "God can use me whether I'm disabled or not. I can praise Him. My faith in Him helps me and others. My faith or spirituality is part of a three legged stool, physical, psychological, and spiritual. Without spirituality I would have done myself in."

It seems that sometimes one of the most powerful ways to bring about change for the person suffering with pain might be the person's spirituality. This might incorporate the person's view of the meaning of the pain or suffering in life. It may involve the person's relationship with God. This concept was expressed by a patient who stated that his "relationship with God" was an "extremely powerful aspect of surviving." He said that God was "an extremely powerful ally in dealing with chronic pain."

"God, please take control." This was the prayer of a thirty-two year old father and his wife when she had a stroke two weeks after giving birth to their third child. Even after the woman was improving clinically, a neurosurgeon consulted and felt that she needed a craniotomy to prevent brain damage due to possible brain swelling that he could see on CT scan. It was terrifying and the father felt completely out of control. This prayer, evidence of a strong faith, was helpful to all who were there. This faith, this prayer, changed the thinking and feelings of all involved.

For many people, connection with God and spirituality are central to their lives. One's spirituality and faith can provide meaning and purpose to life. Do people have a biological predisposition to spirituality or faith? Is the brain or brain/body wired for relationship to God?

In many ways this aspect of our being might encompass all the above treatment approaches. It might give one courage and endurance as one struggles with systematic desensitization and constraint induced movement therapy. It can become an all encompassing change in the salience landscape and emotion regulation. One's relationship with God can utilize mirror neuron systems as one re-learns to help others and learns to ask for help and accept help as well. This aspect of life can be calming, give one a sense of support, and facilitate structure in daily activities.

In terms of pain rehabilitation, this whole concept can bring about a healing epiphany in the person's life. It can help a person change from one who is only focused on pain and lessening of pain to one who is focused more on improving life.

Victor Frankl, holocaust survivor and psychiatrist, in his book, *Man's Search for Meaning*, described a system of psychotherapy called "Logo Therapy." This is a form of existential therapy, which helps persons who are suffering to find meaning and purpose in the experiences, or even to make meaning and purpose out of these life experiences. It is a form of therapy that asks larger questions about why things are the way they are. Understanding the answers, at least to a degree, might be even more healing than changing the situation or fixing the medical problem.

As a person of Christian faith, I speak from the Christian perspective. However, these ideas may also apply to people of many other faiths or no faith at all. We all seem to be on a journey, traveling through the years and decades, experiencing and accomplishing many things in many ways and in many relationships. From my Christian perspective it seems that music, meditations, bible verses, parables, and life stories and experiences can help me and others to understand the journey and help me experience and express more fully the essence of who I am. One's spirituality can help answer the deeper and larger questions, not just about our pain, but more importantly, about our lives.

Calming The Sympathetic Nervous System

Calming the sympathetic nervous system can help lessen pain. When a person is heard, believed, cared for, validated, and feels a sense of support, the sympathetic nervous system is calmed. When the person does not feel abandoned or alone, and feels a sense of teamwork with their care providers, the sympathetic nervous system is calmed. When humor, love, peace, and hope are stimulated, the sympathetic nervous system is calmed. When the person has better understanding about what is really causing the problems and the pain, there is less fear of the unknown and the sympathetic nervous system is calmed. When the person knows more about what to do and what to expect, the sympathetic nervous system is calmed. When the person learns tools and skills to participate in life in a healthy and balanced manner, the sympathetic nervous system is calmed.

The following calm the sympathetic nervous system:

1. Sense of support, validation, caring, compassion

2. Sense of structure and purpose in life activities

3. Appropriate knowledge and information

4. Humor, love, peace, hope

5. Use of healthy, balanced living tools

In contrast, the following activate and prime the sympathetic nervous system, which is not calming:

1. Sense of invalidation, criticism

2. Sense of lack of purpose and lack of structure

3. Confusion, misinformation, fear of the unknown

4. Anger, depression, anxiety, despair

All the mechanisms of pain and suffering, peripheral, central, autonomic are different from person to person. All the mechanisms change from moment to moment depending on the environment, both external and internal. What we do, how we think, what we eat, how we sleep, and with whom we associate all have effects on these mechanisms of pain and the suffering experience. Some people react strongly to changes. Some people notice effects but are not troubled. Some might focus on the pain and stress, while others may not. All of this can vary from person to person and moment to moment. What calms one part of the nervous system may stimulate or activate another part of the nervous system. If you can learn new things and practice new things, maybe you can make a significant difference in your long-term painful experience.

What to Expect; Concluding Remarks:

When the writing of this book began, there was a section on what is normal and it was titled: *Normal, How It All Works*. This was too ambitious and actually impossible to accurately write and describe since no one really knows *how it all works*. The next section of the book was *Abnormal, What Could Go Wrong* and was also too much to deal with. This was also very complicated and misunderstood. What is written now is an effort to describe some of these things in layman's terms. A third section on *What Can Be Done About It* was also complex and incomplete. It too was an attempt to put some very interesting ideas into a workable perspective. Now the whole book is an attempt to give the person who is suffering with chronic pain some understanding of what is normal and abnormal, and to give some hope in the whole medical and non-medical process.

This final section on *What To Expect* is more clear and direct. You can expect to feel somewhat better by knowing and understanding some of this information. This information can help you to be the leader of your team of care providers. It can help you to be a co-manager of your pain. You can become a partner with your doctor and therapists. You can expect to gain more realistic tools, benefits, and hope with respect to the pain and suffering and the whole situation. If you apply some of these concepts diligently to your daily life, you can expect to lessen your pain, anger, depression, anxiety, and improve your sleep, relationships, work, and enjoyable activities. What could be wrong with all of that?

You cannot expect to be cured. If you have a long-term pain problem, a chronic pain problem, possibly a permanent pain problem, this book most likely will not make it go away. However, what you do about it can change it. It does not have to remain the same for the rest of your life. Things can improve.

I don't know if the Dalia Lama's comment is totally true. He said, "Pain is a normal part of life, but suffering is optional." At least to a degree, there is truth in this statement. How you perceive and respond to your situation can make a difference. If you let yourself catastrophize and become significantly emotionally dysregulated, you will feel worse. If you don't let yourself feel any emotions at all, you will be worse as well. Your brain/body knows what is going on and, at least in part, what you need to do about it. Pay attention to your subconscious and your *feelings*, at least a little. *Think* things through as well. Be in charge of your *behaviors* and your rehabilitation as much as you can.

Glossary

A-beta fibers Small, significantly myelinated sensory fibers that transmit non-painful information. *48, 52, 57, 68.*

A-delta fibers Small, slightly myelinated sensory fibers that transmit nociceptive (painful) information particularly about cold and pressure. *9, 41, 48.*

Acetylcholine Neurotransmitter in the central and peripheral nervous systems. *29, 33.*

Action Potential Electrical message traveling down an axon. *28, 32, 79.*

Addiction An uncontrollable compulsion to repeat a behavior regardless of its negative consequences. *3, 155, 175, 198.*

Adrenal Glands Triangle-shaped glands located on top of the kidneys. The outer part, the cortex, produces steroid hormones such as cortisol, testosterone, and aldosterone. The inner part, the medulla, produces epinephrine and norepinephrine, commonly called adrenaline and noradrenaline. When the glands produce too much or too little hormone, you can become ill. *93, 117, 119-125.*

Agonist Drug that attaches to a receptor and has actions that mimic or potentiate those of an endogenous transmitter. *65.*

Allodynia Pain resulting from a stimulus which would normally not cause pain. *Preface, 59, 63, 67, 69, 73, 131.*

Alzheimer's Degenerative neurological disease involving the hippocampus and cortex. *105.*

Amino Acid An organic compound; one of the twenty building blocks of proteins. *19, 20, 29, 36, 39, 41.*

AMPA One type of Glutamate receptor. *Glossary only.*

Amygdala Brain structure associated with emotional memories. *55, 93-104, 113-116, 123-126, 129, 136, 140, 159, 161, 167, 170, 187, 189.*

Angular Gyrus This brain part is an associative area or an area that sits at the intersection or junction of the brain's vision, hearing, and touch centers. It helps bind together the various experiences. *181.*

Antagonist Drug that attaches to a receptor and blocks the action of either an endogenous transmitter or an agonistic drug. *65.*

Anterior Cingulate Cortex (ACC) Front part of the cingulate cortex which is part of the frontal lobe and the limbic system for emotion regulation and executive functions. *Preface, 7, 55, 63, 93, 131-142, 167, 178, 179, 187, 189, 198.*

Anterograde Amnesia Loss of memory for events that happened after brain injury. *110*.

Anticonvulsant Drug that blocks or prevents epileptic convulsions. Some anticonvulsants are also used to treat certain non-epileptic psychiatric disorders. Some anticonvulsants are used to treat certain types of pain, particularly neuropathic pain. *24*.

Antidepressant Drug that is useful in treating mentally depressed patients. *24, 32-34, 170*.

Antipsychotic Drugs that are used to treat patients who may have typical thought disorders; used to calm psychotic states. *Glossary only*.

Antisocial Personality Disorder See Personality Disorders. See Cluster B Disorders. Irresponsible disregard for and violation of the rights of others. *101, 159*.

Anxiety State of uneasiness of mind and apprehension. *Many pages throughout the book*.

Anxiolytic Drug use to relieve symptoms of anxiety. Classically, refers to benzodiazepines and related drugs. *24, 99, 100*.

Asperger's An autism spectrum disorder characterized by significant difficulties in social interaction, and restricted and repetitive patterns of behavior and interests. *149*.

Associativity Pairing a weak input or stimulus with a strong input or stimulus. *80, 82, 84*.

Astrocytes Star shaped glial cells that help form the myelin sheath around the axons of neurons. *23*.

ATP (Adenosine-triphosphate) A nucleotide (building blocks of RNA or DNA) that performs many essential roles in the cell. It is the major energy currency of the cell. *35, 38*.

Attention Deficit Hyperactivity Disorder (ADHD) Learning and behavioral dysfunction characterized by reduced attention span and hyperactivity. *Glossary only*.

Autism A spectrum of neuropsychiatric disorders characterized by deficits in social interaction and communication. *182, 184, 185*.

Autonomic Nervous System Often considered to be part of the peripheral nervous system that controls or regulates the visceral and automatic functions of the body such as heart rate and blood pressure. *52, 53, 61, 73, 78, 146, 147, 155, 184, 185*.

Autonomic Sensitivity Syndrome Hypersensitivity and hyperreactivity of the autonomic nervous system.

Avolition Psychological state characterized by general lack of desire, drive, or motivation to pursue meaningful goals. *42*.

Avoidant Personality Disorder See Personality Disorders. See Cluster C Disorders. Hypersensitivity to potential rejection, humiliation, or shame. *161*.

Axon Nerve cell filament or process that projects electrical impulses away from the cell body. *21, 22, 27-29, 31, 32, 48, 49, 51, 59, 79-81, 87.*

Axon Hillock Area of origin of the axon from the nerve cell body. Initiates the propagation of the action potential down the axon. *22, 27, 28.*

Axon Terminals (Terminal buttons) Somewhat enlarged, often club-shaped endings of the axon fibers. This is on the pre-synaptic side of the synapse, where the message is sent by neurotransmitters to the post-synaptic cell. *22, 28, 29, 59.*

Basal Ganglia Part of the brain that contains large numbers of synapses that use dopamine. It forms part of the extrapyramidal system. Parkinson's disease follows dopamine loss due to neuron loss in this structure. *Glossary only.*

BDNF (Brain Derived Neurotrophic Factor) A protein that is increased in amount in the hippocampus with extended use of antidepressant medications and approaches, and voluntary exercise. Thought to facilitate increased synaptic strength and neurogenesis. *35, 38.*

Benzodiazepines Family of psychoactive drugs used therapeutically to produce sedation, relieve anxiety and muscle spasms, and prevent seizures. *99-101, 153.*

Bipolar Disorder Affective disorder characterized by alternating periods of mania and depression. Also referred to as manic-depressive illness. *100.*

Blood-Brain Barrier The mechanism that keeps many chemicals out of the brain. *23, 24.*

Borderline Personality Disorder (BPD) See Personality Disorders. See Cluster B Disorders. Instability in self-image, interpersonal relationships, mood. *159, 160, 193.*

Bradykinin Peptide that dilates blood vessels and stimulates pain receptors. *35, 37.*

Capillaries Very small blood vessels, intermediary to arteries (bring blood away from the heart) and veins (bring blood to the heart). *23, 36, 37.*

Causalgia See Reflex Sympathetic Dystrophy and Complex Regional Pain Syndrome (CRPS Type II). A condition characterized by pain and tenderness associated with vasomotor instability, skin changes, and development of bony demineralization. Causalgia refers to a more specific definable nerve lesion. *Glossary only.*

Central Nervous System (CNS) Brain and spinal cord. That part of the nervous system housed by bone, the skull and the vertebral column, respectively. *50, 52, 56, 59, 67, 72, 73, 143, 147, 155.*

Central Sensitivity Syndrome Hypersensitivity and hyperreactivity of the brain and spinal cord neurons and networks. *143, 147.*

Cerebral Cortex Extensive outer layer or surface of the brain or gray matter, essentially unmyelinated. *78.*

C-fibers Unmyelinated, slow transmitting, pain message transmitting fibers in the peripheral nervous system. *52, 61, 68.*

Chronic Pain Syndrome Long-term pain that disrupts many aspects of a person's life including work, recreational activities, sleep, relationships, emotions, thinking, chemical use, etc. *Forwar, 145..*

CGRP (Calcitonin Gene Related Peptide) One of the most abundant peptides produced in both peripheral and central neurons. It is the most potent peptide vasodilator and can function in the transmission of pain. *35, 38.*

Cholecystokinin (CCK) Hormone released by the duodenum in response to food distention. *102.*

Chronic Fatigue Syndrome (CFS) Long-term fatigue and exhaustion with no clear underlying identifiable pathology. *141.*

CIPA (Congenitally Insensitive to Pain and Anhidrosis) Very rare genetic biological condition in which the person does not feel pain and has absent or deficient secretion of sweat. *Glossary only.*

Circadian Rhythms Daily rhythmic activity cycle exhibited by many organisms. *Glossary only.*

Cluster A Personality Disorders A cluster of personality disorders whose descriptive characteristics include idiosyncratic thinking, suspiciousness, social withdrawal. These disorders are also called "odd". *158.*

Cluster B Personality Disorders A cluster of personality disorders whose descriptive characteristics include intense emotional experience and expression, poor impulse control, poor frustration tolerance, and mood swings. These disorders are also called "dramatic". *158, 159.*

Cluster C Personality Disorders A cluster of personality disorders whose descriptive characteristics include anxious, worried, emotionally constricted, dependent, and excessive avoidance of pain. These disorders are also called "anxious". *158, 160.*

Codeine Sedative and pain relieving agent. Structurally related to morphine but less potent. *Glossary only.*

Complex Regional Pain Syndrome (CRPS Type I) A condition characterized by pain and tenderness associated with vasomotor instability, skin changes, and development of bony demineralization. Type 1 refers to no specific definable nerve lesion. *145.*

Complex Regional Pain Syndrome (CRPS Type II) A condition characterized by pain and tenderness associated with vasomotor instability, skin changes, and development of bony demineralization. Type II refers to a specific definable nerve lesion. *145.*

Compulsions Repetitive behaviors or mental acts, the goal of which is to prevent or reduce anxiety or distress, not to provide pleasure or gratification. *150, 151.*

Conditioned Stimulus In classical conditioning this is a previously neutral stimulus that, after repeated association with an unconditioned stimulus, elicits the response effected by the unconditioned stimulus. *127, 128, 134, 135, 171, 172.*

Cooperativity Simultaneous stimulation by two or more axons at the same time. *80, 81, 84.*

Cravings An intense desire for some particular thing. *151, 155, 161.*

Cross Tolerance Condition in which tolerance to one drug results in a lessened response to another drug. *Glossary only.*

Cumulative Trauma Disorder Repetitive overuse of a particular part of the body resulting in injury or damage to that body part. *148.*

Cytotoxicity Degree to which an entity is toxic to a cell. *84.*

Cyclooxygenase An enzyme that is found in most tissues and helps turn some fatty acids into prostaglandins. *38.*

Declarative Memory Refers to memories which can be consciously recalled such as facts and events. *104, 105.*

Decrimation A wave of information traveling across a cell becomes less and less strong as it travels. This is not the action potential information that travels down an axon. *28.*

Demyelinization Destruction, removal, or breakdown of the myelin sheath around axons. *51.*

Dendrite Means "branched like a tree." Thousands of little branches of nerve fibers that pick up information and transmit it into the cell. *21, 27, 31, 79, 83, 87, 89.*

Dependence The state of relying on or needing someone or something for aid, support, or the like. Needs the drug to function normally. *See drug dependence.*

Dependent Personality Disorder (DPD) See Personality Disorders. See Cluster C Personality Disorders. Submissive, clinging, fear of separation. *161.*

Depression Common mental disorder that presents with depressed mood, loss of interest or pleasure, feelings of guilt or low self-worth, disturbed sleep, changes in appetite and energy. *Forward, 3, 11, 33, 61, 87, 90, 95, 100, 112, 134, 153, 174, 191, 193, 198, 203.*

Desensitization Decrease in response over time to a stimulus. *169, 171, 172, 176, 197, 199.*

Differential Diagnosis Listing of all possible causes that might explain a given set of symptoms. *Glossary only.*

Dopamine A catecholamine neurotransmitter, helps control the brain's reward and pleasure centers, and helps regulate movement, emotional responses, attention, and thought clarity. It is found in many animals and has many uses in the human being. *33, 40, 140.*

Dorsal Horn Subdivision of the gray matter of the posterior, back part, of the spinal cord. It receives information from afferent fibers. It is also known as the substantia gelatinosa. *9, 41, 42, 57, 62.*

Dorsal Root Ganglion (DRG) A nodule on the dorsal root that contains cell bodies of neurons in afferent spinal nerves. *8, 9.*

Down Regulation Decrease in the number of cell receptors for a chemical, drug, or other stimulus. Decrease in the receptive capabilities of the cells. *59, 87.*

Drug Dependence State in which the use of a drug is necessary for either physical or psychological well-being. *Glossary only.*

Drug Receptor Specific molecular substance in the cell walls of the brain/ body which when stimulated by a drug causes the cell to react. The interaction produces an effect. *Glossary only.*

Drug Tolerance State of progressively decreasing responsiveness to a drug. *3, 43, 44, 65, 87, 151, 152.*

DSM-IV-TR *Diagnostic and Statistical Manual of Mental Disorders*, Fourth Edition, published by the American Psychiatric Association in 1994. The Text Revision of the Fourth Edition was published in 2000. *101, 151, 160.*

Dynorphin A class of opioid peptides found throughout the central and peripheral nervous systems. *39, 41.*

Emotional Freedom Technique (EFT) a form of alternative psychotherapy that uses tapping on acupuncture points while a patient focuses on a specific traumatic memory. This is said to manipulate energy fields some practitioners associate with the human body. *197, 198.*

Emotion Dysregulation Difficulty controlling or managing emotions. Similar to poor impulse control, poor frustration tolerance, intense emotional experience and expression. *112, 193.*

Endogenous Originating, produced, or growing from within an organism, tissue, or cell. *39, 170.*

Endorphin Naturally occurring pain relieving chemical. It causes endogenous morphine-like activity. *39, 42, 87.*

Enkephalin Naturally occurring protein that causes morphine-like activity. *39, 41.*

Ephaptic Transmission The passage of a neural impulse from one nerve fiber, axon, or dendrite to another through the membranes of the structures next to each other. *52, 62.*

Episodic Memory One of two forms of conscious or declarative memory, episodic and semantic. Memory of information about specific past events that involved the self and occurred at a particular time and place. *104, 105, 125.*

Equi-analgesic Strength of pain relieving ability. Comparisons of some commonly used medications are as follows: *Glossary only.*

COMMON OPIOIDS: CONVERSIONS AND COMMENTS

Percocet 5/325 = Oxycodone 5 mg + Tylenol 325 mg
    (comes in various forms such as 7.5/750, or 10/325, etc.)
Typically lasts 4 hours or so.

Vicodin 5/500 = Hydrocodone 5 mg + Tylenol 500 mg
    (one Vicodin is very slightly weaker than one Percocet in general)
    (comes in various forms such as 7.5/750, or 10/325, etc. Often written as Norco,
which is simply Hydrocodone + Tylenol in various forms)
Typically lasts 4 hours or so.

Vicoprofen 7.5/200 = Hydrocodone 7.5 mg + Ibuprofen 200 mg
    (sometimes used if a person cannot tolerate Tylenol)
Typically lasts 4 hours or so.

Duragesic 25 mcg/hour (transdermal fentanyl patch) = about 10 tablets of Oxycodone or
Hydrocodone per day continuously released across the skin.   One patch is typically used for 72 hours. Actually a person receives a range of medication from 4.5 – 13 Percocet per day, and often on the 3rd day is not getting much medication. Duragesic 50 mcg/hour is about equal to 20 tablets per day.

OxyContin = Continuous release Oxycodone = the same chemical and mg as Oxycodone.
Supposed to last 12 hours but often lasts 8 hours or so.

Methadone = about twice as strong as Oxycodone, mg per mg,
(i.e. 10 mg Methadone = 20 mg Oxycodone)
Typically lasts 6 hours or so.

Morphine = about 2/3 the strength of Oxycodone,
    (i.e. 30 mg Morphine = 20 mg Oxycodone)
    There is short acting, immediate release. There is also long-acting, slow release.

Dilaudid 2 mg = about 10 mg Oxycodone
Typically lasts 4 hours or so.

Excitatory Neurotransmitter Makes the neuron more likely to send the message on. *27, 32, 37, 64, 84.*

External Locus of Control Belief that one's life is determined mainly by sources outside one's self. *86.*

Eye Movement Desensitization Reprocessing (EMDR) A form of psychotherapy that was developed to resolve symptoms resulting from disturbing unresolved life experiences and traumas. It is being used for a number of psychological problems. *197.*

Fibromyalgia "Algia" means pain; "My" refers to muscle; "Fibro" refers to the fibers of the muscles. Therefore, "pain in the fibers of the muscles." In reality, this is a diagnosis of exclusion, meaning nothing else is found. The person hurts all over and is tired all the time. There are typically tender spots in eleven of eighteen different areas of the body. *Forward, Preface, 3, 36, 55, 69, 71, 92, 143, 153, 154.*

Fibro-Fog Trouble with clarity of thinking, memory, judgment, decision making, associated with fibromyalgia. *Glossary only.*

Free Nerve Endings Somatosensory nerve endings that are sensitive to painful stimuli. *45-47, 63-65.*

fMRI (Functional Magnetic Resonance Imaging) A technique for measuring the utilization of oxygen and blood flow to particular brain parts and networks during various brain activities. *96.*

Gamma-Amino-Butyric-Acid (GABA) The most abundant inhibitory amino acid neurotransmitter in the brain. *40, 51.*

Generalized Anxiety Excessive anxiety and worry occurring more days than not for at least six months. *99.*

Glial Cells Non-neuronal cells that maintain homeostasis, form myelin, and provide support and protection for the neurons. *26, 35, 38.*

Glial Sheath Membrane of tissue surrounding structures or groups of cells and made up of parts of the glial cells. *23.*

Glucocorticoid "Long-term stress chemical", a class of steroid hormones, excreted from the cortex or surface of the adrenal glands. *120, 123-126.*

Glutamate The most abundant excitatory amino acid neurotransmitter. *37, 64, 65, 84.*

Glutamitergic Synaptic Transmission Transmission of glutamate across the synapse. *Glossary only.*

Habituation A simple form of learning, in which an animal, after a period of exposure to a stimulus, stops responding. *89, 152.*

Hippocampus Major part of the limbic system in humans and other mammals, involved in formation of new memories, consolidation of short term memory, and spatial organization. *93, 103-115, 123-126, 139, 140, 167, 187.*

Histamine An organic nitrogen compound involved in local immune responses as well as regulating physiological function in the gut, released from mast cells, dilates blood vessels and increases vessel wall permeability. *35-37.*

Histrionic Personality Disorder (HPD) See Personality Disorders. See Cluster B Personality Disorders. Overly gregarious and attention seeking. *159, 160.*

Homeostasis The ability or tendency of an organism or cell to maintain internal equilibrium and stability by adjusting its physiological processes. This is done by the coordinated response of its parts to any situation or stimulus. *126.*

Hormone Chemical released by a cell or gland in one part of the brain/body which travels through the blood stream and effects cells in another area of the brain/body. *18, 32, 115, 119, 120, 121, 123.*

HPA Axis Combined system of neuroendocrine units including the Hypothalamus-Pituitary-Adrenal glands, an example of the brain/body connection; very important in the experience of chronic pain and stress. *123-126.*

Hyperalgesia Extreme sensitivity to pain; greater than normal sensitivity to pain. *38, 44, 47, 53, 67, 73.*

Hyperpathia Clinical symptom/sign of neurological disorder whereby a painful stimulus evokes greater pain than would be expected, i.e. a pin prick feels like a knife. *67, 69, 73.*

Hypnosis An artificially induced altered state of consciousness, associated with heightened suggestibility and receptivity to direction. *132, 197, 198.*

Hypothalamus A portion of the brain that contains a number of small nuclei with a variety of hormonal control functions and regulation of many mind/body connections. *8, 93, 99, 115, 116, 121-124.*

Irritable Bowel Syndrome (IBS) Disorder characterized most commonly by cramping, abdominal pain, bloating, constipation, and/or diarrhea. *141.*

Implicit Memory A type of memory in which previous experiences aid in the performance of a task without necessarily conscious awareness of these previous experiences; sometimes equated to unconscious, procedural, emotional memories. *104, 105.*

Inhibitory Neurotransmitter Makes the neuron less likely to send the message on. *27, 32, 40, 73, 116.*

Insular Cortex The insular cortex is involved in the processing of visceral activity, balance, attention, pain, emotion, verbal and motor information, inputs related to music and eating, and all the five senses. *178.*

Internal Locus of Control Belief that one's life is determined mainly by sources inside one's self. *85.*

Ion Channels Pore-forming membrane protein complexes whose function is to facilitate the diffusion or transfer of ions across cell membranes. *51.*

James-Lange Theory Hypothesis on the origin and nature of emotions. States that a response to a stimulus may come before the emotional content of the experience (i.e. a stimulus like seeing a snake makes you jump and then you feel the fear; like "ready, fire, aim"). *180.*

Kluver-Bucy Syndrome Damage to the anterior temporal horns or anterior part of the temporal lobes and bilateral amygdala damage. *100.*

Lamina ll Cross-section of the posterior horn of the spinal cord reveals layers of cells that have different functions and receive different inputs from the periphery. Lamina ll is also called the substantia gelatinosa. *41.*

Learned-Shock-Avoidance A process by which an individual learns a behavior or response to avoid a stressful or unpleasant situation or stimulus (such as a shock). *99.*

Limbic System The complex set of structures that lies deep in the brain and is quite involved with emotions and motivations. Some of the structures, and related structures, include the amygdala, hippocampus, hypothalamus, cingulate cortex, fornix, septum, basal ganglia, ventral tegmental area, and pre-frontal cortex. *55, 56, 77, 78, 95, 104, 115, 133, 139, 159, 161, 184-186.*

Locus Coeruleus A bluish area, nucleus, of the brain stem with many norepinephrine-containing neurons. *40-42.*

Long-Term Depression (LTD) Persistent weakening of synaptic strength and activity. *87, 89, 91, 93.*

Long-Term Potentiation (LTP) Persistent increase in synaptic strength following repetitive stimulation. *79-81, 83, 85.*

Mast Cells Cells found in connective tissue that releases substances such as heparin and histamine; important in immune system responses. *36.*

Memory Consolidation Process by which recent memories are crystallized into long-term memory. *105-110, 126.*

Molecular Consolidation Referring to learning and memory, these are the changes that happen at the molecular level. *106.*

Moro reflex The startle reflex in infants, an involuntary response that is present at birth and usually disappears between the ages of 3 to 6 months. *101.*

Mu-opioid receptors (μ-opioid receptors) These are a class of opioid receptors with high affinity for enkephalins and beta-endorphins but low affinity for dynorphins. *41, 42.*

Muscle Memory A form of procedural memory, motor learning, that involves consolidating a specific motor task into memory through repetition. *106.*

Myelin Sheath The insulating envelope of fatty tissue that surrounds the axon of a nerve cell and facilitates the transmission of nerve impulses. *51.*

Narcissistic Personality Disorder (NPD) See Personality Disorders. See Cluster B Personality Disorders. Grandiosity, arrogance, entitlement, exploitation. *159, 160.*

Narcotics Definition per the United States Drug Enforcement Administration (DEA). The term "narcotic," derived from the Greek word for stupor, originally referred to a variety of substances that dulled the senses and relieved pain. Today, the term is used in a number of ways. Some individuals define narcotics as those substances that bind at opiate receptors (cellular membrane proteins activated by substances like heroin or morphine) while others refer to any illicit substance as a narcotic. In a legal context, narcotic refers to opium, opium derivatives, and their semi-synthetic substitutes. For the purposes of this discussion, the term narcotic refers to drugs that produce morphine-like effects. *39, 42.*

Neocortex The newer, in terms of evolution, portion of the cerebral cortex, showing the most highly evolved stratification and organization and responsible for higher level cognitive functions, such as language, learning, memory, and complex thought. *77, 78, 95.*

Nervi –Nervorum Small nerve filaments innervating the sheath of a larger nerve. *53.*

Networks Parts of the nervous system, brain/body connections, that interact with each other. *Preface, 2, 5, 8, 11, 17, 27, 41, 45, 57, 63, 71, 73, 78, 81, 85, 93, 95, 99, 101, 104, 106, 111, 114, 124, 133, 134, 136, 139, 140, 150, 179-189, 198.*

Neurogenesis Creation of new neurons or birth of new neurons. Most prevalent during pre-natal development, but in some parts of the brain, particularly the hippocampus, it goes on all through life. *85, 139.*

Neurogenic Inflammation Inflammation caused by an injurious stimulus of afferent nerves. *52.*

Neuroma A growth or tumor of nerve tissue. *51.*

Neuron The functional unit of the nervous system. The main cells of the nervous system. *Many references.*

Neuropathic Pain Pain that results from lesion, disease, injury to the somatosensory nervous system. *Many references.*

Neuroplasticity The brain's natural ability to form new connections in order to compensate for injury or even normal changes in one's internal or external environment. *57, 85, 190.*

Neurotransmitters Endogenous chemicals which transmit signals from one neuron to the next neuron or the target cell across a synapse. *17, 19, 21, 23, 29-33, 39, 59, 83, 87, 89, 189.*

NGF (Nerve Growth Factor) Small protein that induces the survival and proliferation of neurons. It is important for the growth and maintenance of many neurons. *35, 38.*

Nitric Oxide A molecule consisting of one atom of nitrogen and one atom of oxygen, and produced by many cells in the body. This is a gas that can act as a retrograde neurotransmitter. *83.*

Nitrous Oxide Commonly known as laughing gas or sweet air. *Glossary only.*

NMDA One type of Glutamate receptor. *64, 65, 67.*

Nociceptive Pain (Somatic, Visceral) Pain experienced due to stimulation of pain receptors by any of the mechanical, chemical, thermal, or any other potentially tissue damaging painful stimuli. Somatic refers to the body in general. Visceral refers to the internal organs, particularly the abdominal cavity. *71, 72.*

Nociceptors Sensory receptors for mechanical, chemical, thermal, or any other potentially tissue damaging painful stimulus. *35-37, 46, 47, 53.*

Norepinephrine (Also called noradrenalin) Catecholamine, hormone and neurotransmitter, with multiple roles in the brain/body including decreased pain and increased energy. *33, 40, 42, 119.*

Nuclei Brain parts or groups or clusters of neurons that all seem to have the same functions, and work together. *27, 111, 115, 136.*

Nucleus Accumbens An area deep in the brain that is an important part of the reward system, emotional learning, operant conditioning. *140.*

Obsessive-Compulsive Disorder (OCD) An Axis I anxiety disorder that includes obsessions and compulsions. *133.*

Obsessive-Compulsive Personality Disorder (OCPD) See Personality Disorders. See Cluster C Personality Disorders. Perfectionism and inflexibility. *145.*

Obsessions Persistent ideas, thoughts, impulses, or images that are experienced as intrusive and inappropriate and that cause marked anxiety or distress. *150, 151.*

Opioids Chemicals that bind to opioid receptors in the brain/body and are typically analgesic or pain relieving. *39-44, 65, 67, 70, 89, 92, 113, 147, 152-156, 166, 188.*

Panic Attacks (PA) Discrete episodes in which there is sudden onset of intense apprehension, fearfulness, or terror, often associated with feelings of impending doom. During these attacks, symptoms such as shortness of breath, palpitations, chest pain or discomfort, choking or smothering sensations, and fear of "going crazy" or losing control may be present. *Preface, 69, 99.*

Panic Disorder (PD) Recurrent unexpected panic attacks with or without agoraphobia. *Glossary only.*

Parahippocampal Gray matter cortical cells that surround the hippocampus. *111.*

Paranoid Personality Disorder See Personality Disorders. See Cluster A Disorders. Misinterprets others' actions. *158, 159.*

Peptide String of amino acids in a chain. *18-21, 29, 35, 38, 39, 53.*

Periaqueductal Gray A core of gray matter nervous tissue surrounding the cerebral aqueduct in the midbrain. *7.*

Periodic Limb Movement Disorder A sleep disorder in which the person experiences repetitive or even rhythmic cramping or jerking of the limbs. Another term is nocturnal myoclonus. *141.*

PET (Positron Emission Tomography) A major diagnostic imaging modality used predominantly in determining the presence and severity of cancers, neurological conditions, and cardiovascular disease. *96.*

Peripheral Sensitivity Syndrome Hypersensitivity and hyperreactivity of the peripheral nervous system neurons and networks. *141, 145, 147.*

Personality Disorders See Personality Traits. Traits that markedly deviate from the expectations of the culture and manifest in at least two of the following domains: cognition, affectivity, interpersonal functioning, impulse control. They are inflexible and pervasive, and cause clinically significant distress or impairment in social, occupational, or other important domains. They are not better accounted for by another mental disorder, and they are not due the direct physiological effects of chemicals or medical problems. *157.*

Personality Traits Enduring patterns of perceiving, relating to, and thinking about the environment and oneself, exhibited in a wide range of social and personal contexts, generally recognizable in adolescence or early adulthood. *156, 157.*

Phantom Limb Pain Pain appearing to come from where an amputated limb used to be. *Glossary only.*

Phobias Type of anxiety disorder. A strong, irrational fear of something that poses little or no actual danger, persistent fear of certain situations, activities, animals, people or other things. *99, 147, 149.*

Pituitary Gland The pituitary gland is a pea-sized endocrine gland located at the base of the brain. The pituitary helps control the release of hormones. *93, 116, 117, 121-124.*

Place Cells Neurons in the hippocampus that exhibit a high rate of firing whenever an animal is in a specific location in an environment. *111.*

Polypeptide About 100 amino acids in a chain. *20, 21.*

Pons The midsection of the brain stem. Just below the midbrain, and just above the medulla. *40, 101, 129.*

Post-synaptic A synapse is a space where biochemical connection between two neurons occurs. Post-synaptic refers to the receiving side of the message or signal. *59, 65, 83, 87, 89.*

Post Traumatic Stress Disorder Flashback or intrusive recollections and nightmares or dreams about a particular trauma. The person experienced, witnessed, or was confronted with an event or events that involved actual or threatened death or serious injury, or threat to the physical integrity of self or others. The person's response involved intense fear, helplessness, or horror. *102.*

Pre-Frontal Cortex Most anterior or front part of the brain. It plays an important role in cognitive control, in the ability to orchestrate thought, action, and self-control. *98.*

Premotor Cortex An area of the brain where neurons are critical in the sensory guidance of movements, intentions with respect to movements, and involvement in selection and choosing of movements. *177, 178.*

Pre-synaptic A synapse is a space where biochemical connection between two neurons occurs. Pre-synaptic refers to the sending side of the message or signal. *27, 59, 83.*

Primary Afferent Fibers Primary means first. Afferent means carrying to or toward. Therefore these are nerve fibers that are the first to carry messages to or toward the central nervous system. *48, 49, 53.*

Procedural Memory This is a most basic and primitive form of memory. It involves how to perform different actions and skills. Much of this is on a subconscious level. *104, 105, 111.*

Prostaglandins Lipid hormone like compounds produced by the body and are responsible for inflammatory features, such as swelling, pain, stiffness, redness and warmth. *38, 53.*

Protein Greater than 200 amino acids in a chain; sometimes many thousands. For example, the millions of receptors embedded in the cell membranes are typically clumps of protein. Some neurotransmitters are proteins as well. Proteins are involved in all cell functions. Some provide structural support, while others are involved in movement. Some are antibodies, enzymes, or hormones, and some help transport other chemicals through the brain/body. *20, 27, 41, 51, 106.*

Psychoactive Drugs or chemical substances that cross the blood-brain barrier and affect brain functioning, causing changes in behavior, mood and/or consciousness. *23, 24.*

Raphe Magnus Nucleus Serotonergic neurons represent the major cell type, about 15–20 percent of the neurons in this nucleus. It is located in the brain stem and sends serotonin throughout the nervous system. *40, 41.*

Receptors At the cellular level they are proteins mainly on the surface of the cells that, when stimulated by neurotransmitters, cause the cell to do something. At the larger, macroscopic level, there are many types of small organs in most tissues and places in the brain body that are sensitive to various types of stimuli. *Many references.*

Referred Pain Patterns Pain felt in one part of the brain/body due to pathology in a different part of the brain/body, such as a heart attack causing left arm pain. There are no nerves directly from the heart to the left arm. However, nerves from the heart and nerves from the left arm go to essentially the same place in the spinal cord. When the message gets up to the brain, the brain may not know where the pain is really coming from. *Glossary only.*

Reflex Sympathetic Dystrophy (RSD) See Complex Regional Pain Syndrome. RSD is an older term. There are several other terms. Condition characterized by pain, tenderness, skin changes, possibly bone demineralization in an affected body part. *84.*

REM (Rapid Eye Movements) Noted when a person is asleep and dreaming.

108.

Repetitive Overuse Syndrome Repetitive, excessive use of a body part resulting in pain and other symptoms; repetitive strain or repetitive stress; often work related; often orthopedic or musculoskeletal. *145.*

Reptilian Complex Brain stem, basal ganglia, cerebellum. American physician and neuroscientist, Paul D. MacLean, originally formulated in the 1960s and advocated its use at length in his 1990 book, *The Triune Brain in Evolution*. The triune brain consists of the reptilian complex, the paleomammalian complex or limbic system, and the neomammalian complex or neocortex, viewed as structures sequentially added in the course of evolution. *77.*

Restless Leg Syndrome Syndrome characterized by an irresistible urge to move one's body (legs) to stop uncomfortable or odd sensations. *141, 155.*

Retrograde Amnesia Loss of memory for events that occurred before brain injury. *110.*

Reticular Activating System In the core of the brain stem. Helps facilitate wakefulness and alertness. *55.*

Retrograde Neurotransmitters Released from the post-synaptic neuron, sent back to and received by the pre-synaptic neuron. *59, 83.*

Retrograde Transmission Process of neurotransmitter release by a post synaptic cell under extensive stimulation, that travels back to the pre-synaptic cell to modify it. *83, 87, 89.*

Re-uptake Reabsorption of a neurotransmitter by the presynaptic terminal. *32, 34.*

Schizoid Personality Disorder See Personality Disorders. See Cluster A Disorders. Indifferent to others' actions. *158, 159.*

Schizotypal Personality Disorder See Personality Disorders. See Cluster A Disorders. Peculiarities of ideation, appearance, and behavior, and deficits in interpersonal relatedness. *158, 159.*

Semantic Memory One of two forms of declarative or conscious memory, episodic and semantic. Semantic memory has to do with meanings, concepts, knowing about things such as knowing what is a cat or a chair. *104, 111.*

Sensitization Increase in response to a stimulus as a result of previous exposure to the stimulus. Sometimes thought of as an increase in response to a mild stimulus as a result of previous exposure to a stronger stimulus. *50, 65, 73, 84, 152.*

Septum Part of the limbic system. Plays a role in reward and reinforcement. Has a key role in inhibiting aggression. *Glossary only.*

Serotonin A monoamine neurotransmitter biochemically derived from tryptophan, primarily found in the gastrointestinal tract, platelets, and the nervous system; its various functions include the regulation of mood, appetite, sleep, and muscle contraction. *33-35, 40-42.*

Shaping Modifies behavior by reinforcing behaviors that progressively approximate the target behavior (operant response). *191.*

Soma Cell body. *Many references.*

Somatoform Disorder Physical symptoms that suggest a general medical condition, but not fully explained medically, and not the result of substance use or another mental disorder. *Glossary only.*

Spaced Repetition A learning technique that incorporates intervals of time between subsequent review and practice of material to be learned. *107.*

Specificity Refers to specific active synapses and the results of repetitive active stimulation at these synapses. If some of the synapses onto a cell have been highly active, and others have not been active, only the active ones become strengthened. If you practice a measure of piano music over and over in a particular or specific way, then this is what you will learn. If you experience pain and practice only specific thoughts, feelings, behaviors, then this will become your expertise. *80, 81.*

Spectrum Disorders Disorders that seem to be very similar to each other, or at least have very similar characteristics; some examples might include "schizophrenia spectrum disorders" which involve a number of different thought disorders, "affective spectrum disorders" which involve a number of mood disorders, and "autistic spectrum disorders" which involve a number of different types and presentations of autism. *Glossary only.*

Spinothalamic Tract Sensory pathway originating in the spinal cord. It transmits information to the thalamus about pain, temperature, itch and touch. *55.*

Stress Diathesis Psychological model which explains behavior as the result of two factors: biological factors including genetic pre-disposition or vulnerability, and internal and external environmental or situational stresses. *158.*

Synapse Small gap between the neurons. Allows for chemical message to transmit from one side of the gap to the other side. *22, 28-32, 59, 64, 79-81, 87, 106.*

Startle Response Complicated involuntary reaction to a sudden unexpected stimulus and involves flexion of most skeletal muscles and a variety of visceral and neurological reactions. This is mainly a survival mechanism. *102.*

Steroids Five classes of hormones including estrogens, progestins, androgens, glucocorticoids, and mineralocorticoids. These have many different functions in the brain/body. *123.*

Substance P Neurotransmitter that is released by nerves that are sensitive to pain. *35, 36, 38, 42, 53, 59, 68.*

Substantia Gelatinosa A narrow, dense, vertical band of gelatinous gray matter forming the dorsal part of the posterior column of the spinal cord. Involved in the experience of nociceptive and thermal primary afferent inputs. *4, 56.*

Supplementary Motor Area Key in planning of behaviors and movements. *8, 177, 178.*

Sympathetically Maintained Pain Pain that is associated with problems or abnormalities in the sympathetic nervous system. *62.*

Thalamus An area deep in the brain that helps to process and relay movement and sensory information. It is like a relay station for the brain/body, which takes in sensory information from different parts of the body and passes this information on to the cerebral cortex. It has many other functions including regulation of wakefulness and sleep. *9, 55, 187.*

Tolerance State of progressively decreasing responsiveness to a drug. Tolerance can occur to other stimuli as well. *See Drug Tolerance.*

Unmyelinated Without a myelin sheath. *48-51, 57, 68.*

Urbach-Weithe Disease Rare genetic disorder resulting in calcification and wasting away of the amygdala. *101.*

Vasovagal Syncope Most common cause of fainting. Vasovagal syncope occurs when the body overreacts to triggers, such as the sight of blood or extreme emotional distress. A brief loss of consciousness caused by a sudden drop in heart rate and blood pressure, which reduces blood flow to the brain. *92.*

Ventral Posterior Thalamus Area of the thalamus that receives somatosensory information. An area of the thalamus where the convergence of sensory information occurs. *8.*

Wind-up Repetitive stimulation of the peripheral nerve with the intensity sufficient to activate the pain sensitive fibers leads to a progressive build-up of the magnitude of electrical response in the spinal cord. Thus, repeated strong messages from the peripheral nerves build-up the electrical responses in the spinal cord. The spinal cord becomes more sensitive and more reactive, more ready to receive messages from the periphery, and more ready to send messages up to the brain. *62, 66.*

Withdrawal Many uncomfortable symptoms that might occur as the result of discontinuation of addicting substances or behaviors. *3, 113, 147, 149, 151-156.*

ABOUT THE AUTHOR

Jay Tracy, PA-C, PsyD, LP, has been a Physician Assistant since 1975. He is a Licensed Psychologist with a doctorate in clinical psychology. He has a BA in Psychology, a BA in Physiology, a BS in Allied Health, and is an RN. He has worked at Courage Center in the Chronic Pain Rehabilitation Program and Phoenix Center Pain Services in Golden Valley since 2005. Previously, he worked at Sister Kenny Institute, Abbott Northwestern Hospital Chronic Pain Program for six years. Prior to this, he was the Director of a Chronic Pain Program and Back and Neck Rehabilitation Program at The Minneapolis Clinic of Neurology for twenty-seven years. He also worked in Neurosurgery at the Veterans Administration Hospital. He is an adjunct professor at Bethel University, teaching neuropsychology to graduate students in counseling psychology. He is the author of the book, *"Pain: It's Not All In Your Head; The Test Don't Show Everything."* He is a member of the American Academy of Physician Assistants and past-president and fellow member of the Minnesota Academy of Physician Assistants. He is happily married, thirty-six years, has three grown children and five grandchildren. He loves to play the mandolin and other musical instruments and sings in a group at his church.

20434459R00144

Made in the USA
Middletown, DE
26 May 2015